Stefan Ball & Judy Howard

Emotional Healing for Cats

Index by Ann Griffiths
Illustrated by Kate Aldous

SAFFRON WALDEN
THE C.W. DANIEL COMPANY LIMITED

First published in Great Britain in 2000
by The C.W. Daniel Company Limited
1 Church Path, Saffron Walden,
Essex, CB10 1JP, United Kingdom

ISBN 0 85207 336 4

Designed by Jane Norman
Production in association with
Book Production Consultants plc, 25–27 High Street,
Chesterton, Cambridge, CB4 1ND
Typesetting by Cambridge Photosetting Services
Printed and bound by Biddles, Guildford, England.

Emotional Healing for Cats

By the same authors

Judy Howard
The Bach Flower Remedies: Step by Step
Bach Flower Remedies for Women
Growing Up with Bach Flower Remedies

Stefan Ball
Bach Flower Remedies for Men
The Bach Remedies Workbook
The Bach Flower Gardener

Stefan Ball & Judy Howard
Bach Flower Remedies for Animals

Dedication

For Smuts (9th May 1999 – 8th April 2000)

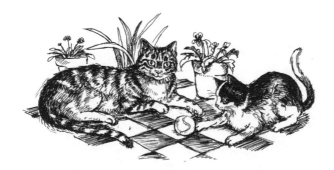

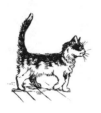

Contents

Introduction

What are cats really like? To people who don't like them all cats are more or less the same – aloof, unsociable and touchy. Or else they are invariably affectionate and playful, or maybe sneaky, cruel and too clever by half.

People love to generalize about cats. Yet the fact that the generalizations vary so widely points to the truth – that cats, like people, are a mixed bunch. Each cat is different, with its own individual personality and individual view of the world. When we get down close and look at the way they feel – about each

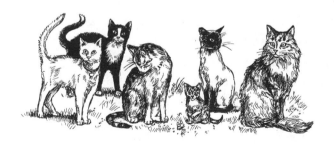

other, about their lives and about us – we can see our own personality types and emotional patterns mirrored in theirs. The triggers for emotions might be different – cats and humans get upset over different things – and we might express our upset in different ways. But the actual upsets – fear, jealousy, impatience, intolerance – these are the same.

This book can help when things go wrong with feline emotions. It draws on the work of a key figure in the history of 20th century medicine, Dr Edward Bach, and shows how to apply his system of 38 emotional medicines to the cat world.

The book is split into three parts. Part One introduces the system. It tells you how to start thinking about your cat's individual personality and moods, how to mix remedies together and when and how to give them. It lists the 38 remedies in full, tells you what each one is for, and gives examples of situations in which you could use them. If you are new to Dr Bach's work the idea of treating negative emotions with medicines might seem strange, and you might find it difficult to see how balancing emotions can affect physical problems like heatstroke or viral infection. We address these questions in Part One, and show how the remedies can benefit cats and their carers.

Part Two lists common feline ailments, offering quick access to the system when your cat is under the weather. First look for the heading that most closely describes the problem that you and your cat are coping with. Then look at the suggested remedies. Once you have found one or two that seem to cover the problem re-read the full remedy indications given in Part One. Cross-checking will help you select the right medicines for your cat's particular emotional state.

Finally, Part Three outlines alternative natural therapies for cats and suggests ways in which you can follow up this introduction to Bach Flower Remedies.

Acknowledgements

We are grateful to Annette Miro-Cassar and Nancy Muller for permission to use their testimonials in the book. And we would like to thank our partners, children, friends and colleagues for all their support and encouragement.

Special thanks are due to Heather Simpson of the Natural Animal Centre, who checked the text at very short notice.

If you have any ideas for improving future editions of this book or would like to tell us about your successes and failures with the remedies, please write to the authors c/o The Bach Centre. The address is in Part Three.

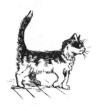

Part One

The Bach Flower Remedies

Dr Edward Bach practised medicine during the early part of the 20th Century. He enjoyed a highly successful career in many branches of the profession and qualified in surgery. But it was during his time as a pathologist that he began to examine the relationship between chronic disease and the immune system. While undertaking extensive research in bacteriology he developed a group of pioneering vaccines which proved successful in treating a number of chronic diseases.

Although this pioneering work brought him international recognition, he dreamed of finding a safer and gentler means of relieving people of their suffering. Homoeopathy offered him many of the answers – it provided a safe, minimal-dose alternative to the concentrated vaccination, and meant that injections were not necessary. The homoeopathic preparations – known as nosodes – could be given orally, and for this reason were less intrusive and painful.

Ever since medical school Dr Bach had made a close study of human nature. Unusually for his time, he was as interested in the fears, worries and hopes of his patients as he was in their physical ailments. He saw them as individuals, with lives that extended beyond the bounds of the hospital ward. He would spend hours listening to what they said and taking note of their individual characters, and noticed that emotional outlook and attitude determined how well they responded to treatment. The state of mind of his patients was crucial to their wellbeing and general state of health.

The first practical application of this insight came when he realised that patients with a particular outlook on life required the same nosode, regardless of their physical complaint. Soon the personality and mood of his patients became the determining factor in diagnosis and prescription. It was not long before Dr Bach dispensed with clinical physical examination altogether.

He then sought to extend his ideas into the search for new treatments. Having established the importance of considering the whole person and not just the disease, he concluded that true healing would only come when he could find a way to treat the patient's state of mind directly. The ideal medicine would have the capacity to heal at the most fundamental level, and so prevent physical disease before it took place.

The search for these new remedies took up the rest of his life. One by one he discovered 38 remedies: 36 prepared from the flowers of wild trees, shrubs and plants, one from a cultivated plant and one from natural healing water. He finished his research in 1935, once the system was complete. Just over a year later, in 1936, he died.

How the remedies work

Each of Dr Bach's remedies treats a specific state of mind or way of thinking. Larch is the remedy for people who lack confidence, and its action is to remove the fear of failure. Gentian gives encouragement to those who have suffered a setback. Clematis is for when we daydream and find it hard to concentrate on the present. Most of the time we feel a mixture of emotions, so when we want to we can mix together individual remedies into hundreds of millions of combinations. This flexibility means that 38 remedies can treat the varied emotional needs of every living thing, making the Bach system unique in its combination of power and simplicity. But how exactly does it work?

We can think of emotional states as vibrations or sound waves. A pure note rings clear, and reflects a positive, healthy emotion such as love, kindness, or joy. The sound of a cracked or muffled note is repressed and distorted, negative and unhealthy – the equivalent of hate, cruelty or despair. The 38 remedies vibrate at the same pitch as the basic positive emotions. Taking the right remedy resonates with the repressed note and helps it ring out clearly and strongly once more. The note sings and the negative distortion disappears.

This is what we mean when we say that the remedies don't put anything into you that isn't there already. A guitar contains all possible pure notes already, but it may not sound out because something is damping down the strings. Putting a tuning fork onto the sound box causes the corresponding string on the guitar to vibrate in sympathy. In the same way taking a remedy calls out the positive quality already inside us and dispels the negative states that hid it.

This theory assumes that particular plants are in some mysterious way related to human beings. Dr Bach certainly believed this, and he was on fairly solid scientific ground when he did so. If you go far enough back in time – 1.8 billion years, according to the sociobiologist Edward O. Wilson – flowering plants and animals, including humans, share the same ancestors. Animals and plants have evolved apart since then, but continue to use the same amino acids and many of the same vitamins and minerals. From New Agers hugging trees to orthodox medicine's traditional and on-going dependence on plants for medicine, much natural and orthodox healing relies on a fundamental spiritual and physical correspondence between plant and animal. We cannot say this proves that plant energies are related to emotions, but it suggests that the idea is not as far-fetched as it might at first appear.

Any scientist will tell you that all this talk of vibrations and sounds is not scientific. We would agree it is a helpful metaphor for energies that science is only just beginning to explore, and we would claim no more for it than that. What is certain is that solid research now supports the relationship between emotions and health. Molecular messengers between emotional states and the immune system have been identified and named. Psychoneuroimmunology – the study of the way the central nervous and immune systems interact – has shown that happiness and positive emotions really do affect physical health, just as Dr Bach claimed. We can only guess what remarkable rediscoveries science will make in the future.

A–Z of the 38 remedies

When you buy remedies you will see that they are numbered from 1 to 38 according to their alphabetical order in English. We have listed them in this same order for easy reference when you are using Part Two of this book.

1. Agrimony

General indication – used to help those who hide their troubles behind a cheerful face.

Cats of this nature may be difficult to identify because you often have to guess at the torture concealed inside an apparently cheerful animal. They will be inclined to be good-natured, happy, peace-loving creatures, and will try to defuse painful situations or potential confrontations by turning them into a game. One indication may be that they are restless when asleep, or seem vaguely agitated yet remain playful and in good humour.

Things to look for:

- ♡ cats that appear happy but develop displacement activities such as spraying in the house.

- ♡ cats that are particularly playful when under stress, or when there is emotional discord in the house.

- ♡ obvious injury or illness accompanied by purring or game-playing.

- ♡ restless sleep and sleeplessness.

2. **Aspen**

General indication – used to treat vague, nameless fears, and feelings of uneasiness and foreboding without there being anything specific to feel anxious about.

Cats in need of Aspen will seem afraid of something that is not really there. Theirs is a free-floating anxiety, not attached to anything specific like a loud noise or strangers, but simply in the air.

Things to look for:

- ♡ cats that seem nervous and anxious in familiar, safe environments.

- ♡ cats that jump and run at every sound, even when the cause of the sound is non-threatening.

- ♡ sudden, unexplained panic.

3. **Beech**

General indication – given to encourage the latent sense of tolerance and understanding in those who are critical and intolerant of other ways of life. Those needing this remedy will believe that their own way of doing things is the only sensible and reasonable one, and that everyone who does things differently is simply stupid.

Cats in a Beech state may turn their noses up if you haven't prepared food in the way they like. They will become irritated quite quickly, and will take the time to let you know of their disapproval. However, under-socialised cats that scratch or wriggle away when you pick them up would do better with the Mimulus remedy.

Things to look for:

♡ cats that behave irritably when their normal living arrangements are disrupted.

♡ cats that show intolerance of new people, foods, animals etc.

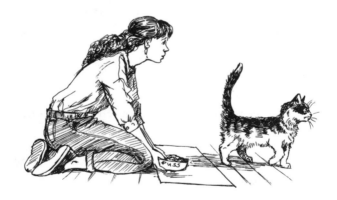

4. Centaury

General indications – used to encourage the willpower of those who are easily dominated. Those needing Centaury will do anything for anyone, are always obliging and ready to serve, but can find it hard to say 'no' and at the extreme fail to live their own lives at all.

Cats of this type are soft and compliant. They don't tend to fight back if they are subject to aggression or attack. They may be timid and introverted, and other animals will find it easy to dominate them.

Things to look for:

♡ cats that are bullied by other cats and cannot seem to respond or escape.

♡ cats that have suffered abuse or cruelty and as a result can't stand up for themselves.

♡ cats that never take the initiative in social interaction.

5. Cerato

General indications – used to strengthen the self-belief of those who do not trust their own instincts, and because of this tend to question their decisions as soon as they have made them. They seek the reassurance of others, hoping for confirmation that they are doing the right thing, and may accept bad advice and so end up doing the wrong thing.

All cats look at cats and people and blink to signal non-aggression and to open a dialogue. Cerato cats will do this to excess, demonstrating their lack of certainty. Even after the event they may look for confirmation that they have acted correctly or appropriately.

Things to look for:

♡ cats that need reassurance even before doing something they are allowed to do, such as playing with a favourite toy or clawing at a scratching post.

6. Cherry Plum

General indications – given to help bring calm and restore sanity to those who feel on the point of losing control, and perhaps committing some violence that they would never do in their right minds.

Cherry Plum is a fear remedy. Just as children are frightened by their own temper tantrums, so cats can be made hysterical and terrified by the intensity of their own emotions. Cherry Plum is the remedy to restore self-possession and remove the fear.

Cherry Plum is also the main remedy for self-mutilation, as seen in cats that bite at their own fur.

Things to look for:

♡ self-injury, especially when sudden or frenzied.

♡ uncontrolled hissing, scratching etc.

♡ cats that panic and do anything to escape, regardless of the risk of injuring themselves.

♡ uncontrolled attacks on kittens or other cats.

7. Chestnut Bud

General indications – used to help those who repeat the same mistakes and do not seem to learn from their errors – or from the example of others.

This remedy can be given to cats that take a long time to learn how life with humans can be made to work. It is not a panacea for any cat that does not do exactly what you want, however – there may be very good reasons why your cat is not learning from you, and if you are making mistakes you might think about taking Chestnut Bud yourself.

Things to look for:

♡ cats that cannot learn simple rules regarding toilet use, scratching etc. despite repeated (and gentle) training.

♡ cats that repeat behaviour despite the bad effects that follow – for example the cat that begs milk from your neighbour despite the fact that it always gets diarrhoea afterwards.

8. Chicory

General indications – used to bring out the positive, generous side of loving individuals who need to be loved in return, and who get upset if they don't get the attention they feel they deserve. Chicory types at their most negative are possessive and emotionally manipulative.

Cats of this type are happiest when they are able to show and receive affection. They may be unwilling to share you and therefore seem possessive when other people or animals are around. They may pine for you when you are not there, making

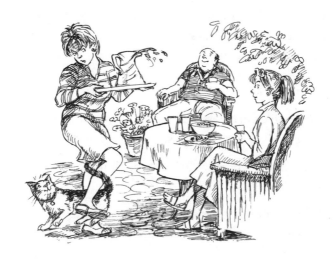

their hurt feelings known through pathetic looks and hurt silences.

Things to look for:

- ♡ cats that are forever under the feet of 'their' humans but show little liking for strangers.
- ♡ cats that guard and shepherd family members (or kittens) to an excessive degree.
- ♡ cats that feign illness to get attention.
- ♡ cats that compete for your attention, either with your other pets, or your children, or with the television etc.

9. Clematis

General indications – used to help ground those who live in dreams of future happiness, so that they can act in the present and make happiness come true now.

Clematis cats seem to fall asleep more easily and more often than their litter-mates. They have little liking for or link with everyday reality, and instead live in a world of their own, not paying attention to what is going on around them any more than they absolutely have to.

Things to look for:

- ♡ excessive sleepiness (remember, however, that the average cat sleeps about sixteen hours a day).
- ♡ cats that get into accidents through not paying attention to where they are.
- ♡ cats that do not notice positive stimuli (like you calling their name, or the sound of food being prepared).

10. Crab Apple

General indications – given to help those who feel ashamed or disgusted at their own appearance, or who feel contaminated, whether by disease, poison or unclean living. Crab Apple types tend to fuss over minor details, particularly related to cleanliness, and have a tendency towards trivial obsessions and compulsive behaviour.

Cats in this state may appear particularly distressed when suffering from skin complaints or parasite infestation. They may groom themselves to excess, or exhibit other forms of obsessive behaviour.

Things to look for:

- ♡ cats that are overly fastidious, for example refusing to use a litter tray that has only been used once before.

- ♡ cats that exhibit compulsive behaviour, such as constantly chasing their own tails or running up and down curtains.

- ♡ cats that groom constantly, even to the extent of doing themselves damage, or that are unable to groom due to physical illness or disability.

- ♡ cats that seem depressed due to parasitic infection, bowel problems etc.

- ♡ depression linked with any skin problem that affects the way the cat looks.

11. Elm

General indications – used to restore a sense of self-assurance to those who have accepted too much responsibility and as a result are suffering from a temporary loss of confidence. In contrast with the Larch state (see below) Elm types know they can do things, but sometimes feel overwhelmed by the sheer number or scale of the things they have to do.

Your normally capable and self-confident cat may seem dejected and down in the mouth when it is in an Elm state. This usually happens when the Elm cat has something new to deal with on top of an already full workload: a nursing mother having to cope with the arrival of noisy house guests, perhaps, or a new human baby upsetting the routine at just the wrong time.

Things to look for:

♥ cats that are struggling to cope with additional pressures or demands, such as the birth of a large litter of kittens or the arrival of a new tom in the neighbourhood.

♥ busy, capable cats that lose their confidence in illness.

12. **Gentian**

General indications – given to those who have suffered a setback of some kind and as a result feel discouraged and despondent. The Gentian state is a mild form of depression, and the remedy gives encouragement so that it can be overcome quickly.

Try Gentian whenever something has gone wrong in your cat's life – whether it is unexpected competition from a new neighbourhood cat or the loss of a favourite toy – and she responds by becoming melancholy.

Things to look for:

♥ cats that respond to setbacks by withdrawing or becoming despondent.

♥ cats that seem inclined to give up easily when they fall ill.

13. Gorse

General indications – this remedy is given to those who have gone a step beyond the Gentian state, and have reached the point where they really have given up. It may be obvious to everyone else what the solution to a problem is, but those in the Gorse state decide that nothing more can be done and drop anchor in a sea of hopelessness.

Cats in this state are very down and seem full of despair. They make no effort to enjoy life or recover from illness. The remedy helps strengthen their natural hope and faith so that they can fight illness more effectively.

Things to look for:

♡ cats that react very badly when things go wrong, and do not respond to encouragement from you.

♡ Gentian cats (see above) that have fallen further down into despair.

♡ cats that have stopped fighting illness and do not try to get better.

14. Heather

General indications – used to widen the perspective of people who are overly wrapped up in their own lives, allowing them to see the needs of others. Those in a negative Heather state cannot bear to be alone and will seek attention from anyone. They enjoy talking about their troubles and people who seem willing to listen find it difficult to get away.

Heather cats will follow anyone who is prepared to give them even the minimum of encouragement. They show no real preference for members of their human family, or for anyone else: any audience will do as long as it is prepared to put up with their demand for company and constant attention.

Things to look for:

- ♡ cats that follow people around, including strangers, and demand attention by jumping onto laps etc.

- ♡ normally quiet cats that become unusually vocal.

- ♡ cats that are with you as much as possible, but do not respond to your calls or signals.

15. **Holly**

General indications – given to encourage the hidden loving heart of those who give way to strong negative feelings about others, such as hatred, suspicion, envy and spite.

Wrongly thought of as being 'the remedy for anger' – there are in fact many possible remedies for anger – Holly is often given to cats inappropriately. It may be indicated if your cat is especially suspicious of strangers or jealous of a newcomer to the family. But if there are symptoms of fear then Mimulus or Rock Rose (see below) would normally be preferred – and in the feline world fear of humans is far more common than spite.

Things to look for:

- ♡ attacks or aggression that go on even after the other cat has given in.

- ♡ aggressive body language and threat towards strangers (but only where fear can be ruled out as a cause).

- ♡ jealous attacks on potential rivals, such as new kittens or new family members.

16. Honeysuckle

General indications – given to help those who live in the past, either reliving past happiness or wallowing in regrets and sad recollections. It helps them enjoy the present more, and renews faith that there is always something in life worth looking forward to.

Signs of a Honeysuckle state in a cat include a lack of attention and a liking for places or activities that it associates with the past or with previous owners. Grieving cats that have lost beloved companions might need this remedy if the grieving process goes on longer than is natural.

Things to look for:

♡ dreaminess and inattention (see also Clematis).

♡ cats that return to former homes or former owners.

♡ failure to thrive in new situations.

♡ homesickness and pining.

17. Hornbeam

General indications – used to give a boost to those who find it difficult to get started, or who feel tired at the mere thought of the tasks ahead. For this reason Hornbeam is often described as the 'Monday morning' remedy.

Look for listlessness and a lack of energy in cats that have rested well and should by rights be full of life. (As in all such cases obtain the advice of a vet in order to ensure that there is no organic reason for the unexplained tiredness.)

Things to look for:

♡ lethargy that seems to wear off as the day goes on.

♡ cats that are reluctant to play but full of energy once
they begin.

♡ reluctance to begin an everyday activity – for
example, cats that sniff around a bowl of their
favourite food, and go and return several times
before starting to eat.

18. **Impatiens**

General indications – given to bring calm and patience to those
who live life in a rush, or who are agitated or irritable when
things go wrong or there is a delay.

Cats in need of Impatiens will always want to be getting on

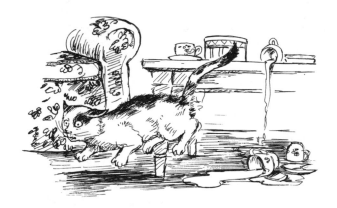

to the next thing, even when the current thing is something
they like or are interested in. They may behave badly if they are
forced to wait for food or to be let out, or if there is any other
delay in their daily routine.

Things to look for:

♡ cats that rush around a lot and are never still.

♡ cats that go from one activity to another very quickly.

♡ reluctance to stay with kittens and other slower or less decisive animals.

♡ frequent mishaps and minor accidents, caused by not taking sufficient time before taking action.

♡ irritability that comes and goes quickly.

19. Larch

General indications – used as a treatment for lack of confidence in those who think they are not good enough and so are bound to fail. This becomes an excuse – sometimes a welcome excuse – not to try things in the first place, or to stop trying at the first setback.

Look for any avoidance of challenges – whether the challenge comes from other cats or from the environment – and a generally unadventurous approach to life. Larch can also be used whenever a cat is going through a particularly difficult task – such as giving birth – and seems to lack the essential self-belief needed to make it a success.

Things to look for:

♡ cats that avoid more dominant cats, noisy children, friendly strangers etc. (see also Mimulus).

♡ cats that are hesitant faced with new situations, foods or environments.

♡ cats that tend to rely on others to make the first move in any encounter.

20. Mimulus

General indications – this is given to those who feel fearful or anxious about something specific. The 'something' can be tangible, such as a particular person, a type of animal or a picture, or it can be something abstract, such as illness or hunger – but in all cases it is something that can be named. Mimulus is also used to help those who tend to be shy and timid, and so find it difficult to interact with others.

The cat in need of Mimulus may appear timid and withdrawn, similar to a Larch or Centaury cat. It may start violently at loud noises or show obvious signs of fear in the presence of whatever it is that it is afraid of.

Things to look for:

♡ fearful body language, such as flattened ears, dilated pupils and arched back.

♡ fear-based aggression, biting, scratching etc.

♡ normally confident cats that attempt to flee specific people or situations, such as the vet or car travel.

♡ cats that jump when there is an unexpected noise.

♡ reluctance to approach strangers, children etc.

21. Mustard

General indications – given to help those who feel unhappy and gloomy, as if their lives were blighted, but who can think of nothing that would justify this feeling. Often all is well in their lives, yet still they feel full of deep melancholy and unhappiness.

Look for obvious signs of depression in your cat, and where there is no event in its life that would justify this consider

Mustard as one possible remedy. (Always get an opinion from the vet in cases of sudden unexplained switches of mood, as these can indicate the presence of organic disease.)

Things to look for:

- ♡ gloom that descends out of the blue, when all environmental conditions seem right.

- ♡ depressed body language or posture.

22. Oak

General indications – used to help those steady and reliable types who because of their great strength fail to understand their own limits. They are capable of amazing feats of endurance, but continue long after they should have rested and in the end may crack under the strain. The remedy has a two-fold action: restoring expended willpower and determination, and teaching restraint and the ability to stop without being broken first.

Oak-type cats are methodical rather than vivacious, more plodders than racers. Their strength is in stamina and reliability. They do not complain even under extreme pressures, but at difficult times you can give them the remedy to help them take better care of themselves.

Things to look for:

- ♡ strong, reliable, steady cats that have a sudden breakdown in health.

- ♡ cats that try to continue their normal routine despite illness and exhaustion.

23. Olive

General indications – this remedy helps restore those who feel exhausted after making some great effort – whether mental, spiritual or physical. It is often contrasted with Hornbeam (see above), which is for tiredness before any effort has been made.

Olive can be used to help cats that are recovering from illness and are exhausted by the process of convalescence.

Things to look for:

♡ exhaustion after a period of activity.

♡ fatigue caused by a struggle against illness or disease.

24. Pine

General indications – given to those who feel guilty about things done or left undone. Even if they have not actually done anything wrong they will take the blame, sometimes excusing the real guilty party in the process.

Pine is often given to cats in error. If you are angry because your cat has clawed your armchair it may be frightened of you and look away or to the side in order to show submission and so appease your anger. You may see this as 'looking guilty' and select Pine, but the cat may not think that it has done anything wrong at all. On the other hand, some cats get nervous when we get angry, even when our anger is actually directed somewhere else. They assume they are responsible, and this in itself can be an indication for Pine. A genuine Pine state can be hard to spot in practice as generally morose and edgy behaviour may be the only evidence you have. You will have to rely on some intelligent guesswork based on your own instincts and assessment of the situation.

Things to look for:

> ♡ submissive behaviour when things happen that do not concern the cat – but examine your own behaviour first, and consider Mimulus for the cat instead of Pine.

25. Red Chestnut

General indications – used to help restore calm and clear-thinking to those who are over-anxious about the well-being of loved ones. They fear something terrible will happen, not to themselves, but to the people they care about.

One sign that this remedy is needed may be over-aggressiveness by a mother cat towards anyone who tries to get near her babies. This is a natural response – but where the concern is exaggerated try Red Chestnut to restore a sense of proportion. (Chicory could also be helpful – see above.)

Things to look for:

> ♡ cats that are constantly moving their kittens from one safe place to another.

> ♡ cats that display fear or fear aggression when anyone approaches kittens.

> ♡ cats that become anxious when their kittens – or you – are out of sight.

> ♡ cats that look out anxiously for the return of beloved humans.

26. Rock Rose

General indications – used to unfreeze those who are in the grip of absolute terror, either at something that is happening to them, or at the sight of something happening to another creature.

In practice it can be difficult to draw a firm line between the cat that needs Mimulus and the one that needs Rock Rose. The key lies in the intensity of the fear: in the Rock Rose state the cat will either be frozen with terror, or will go berserk with fear and attack everything (in which case Cherry Plum has a part to play as well).

Things to look for:

♡ panic.

♡ frozen fear – the cat may actually shiver and feel cold to the touch.

♡ desperate attempts to escape.

♡ desperate attack where there seems no means of escape.

In *Heal Your Cat the Natural Way* holistic vet Richard Allport tells of his use of Rock Rose for one particular cat:

"Bernadette had gone missing. She turned up four weeks later, but kept hiding and refusing food – something had obviously frightened her severely. Giving medication would be difficult but she was drinking, so drops of ... Rock Rose (for panic) and Mimulus (for fear of specific situations) were added to her water ...

"Within a few days, Bernadette was calming down, and soon eating well and enjoying being stroked."

27. Rock Water

General indications – given to encourage mental and emotional flexibility in those who drive themselves hard. Rock Water types set themselves high targets, and gain satisfaction and pleasure from self-denial. They start out with the idea that the end justifies the means – they must suffer in order to achieve perfection – but discipline and self-abnegation quickly become an end in themselves.

Self-denial is not an obvious feline trait, and cats that avoid home comforts like warmth and shelter may need remedies for fear rather than Rock Water. The true Rock Water cat may appear driven to carry out its duties and go on patrolling its territory even when it is tired or ill. Or it may live in a very regimented way, always performing the same actions at the same time and getting upset if it is obliged to break its routine.

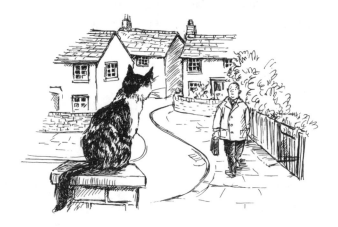

Things to look for:

♡ excessive dislike of changes to an established routine.

♡ regular habits continued despite illness and bad weather.

28. Scleranthus

General indications – used to encourage decisiveness in those who are unable to choose between the options in front of them.

A cat that needs Scleranthus will appear indecisive, sometimes even in trivial matters such as choosing where to take an afternoon nap. Scleranthus is also associated with mood swings and emotional imbalance, and with travel sickness. (Always consult a vet to rule out possible organic causes.)

Things to look for:

- ♡ cats that hesitate when faced with decisions.
- ♡ cats that go from one thing to another and back again, without really settling.
- ♡ mood swings and travel sickness.
- ♡ dizziness, loss of balancing skills and frequent falls – but take your cat to the vet first for a check-up.

29. Star of Bethlehem

General indications – this remedy gives comfort to those suffering from a shock of some kind, or who feel great loss following a sudden bereavement.

Star of Bethelehem is often given to cats rescued from mistreatment or cruelty, and as such is a popular standby treatment in many animal shelters and rescue homes.

Things to look for:

- ♡ cats (especially from rescue homes) that seem to have difficulty adjusting to kind treatment.
- ♡ evidence of past or present mistreatment or trauma.
- ♡ deaths or departures in the close feline or human family.
- ♡ unaccountable changes of character or behaviour following a shock.

Sometimes treating shock can have remarkable repercussions on physical health. Dr Richard Pitcairn gives a good example of this in his 1982 *Complete Guide to Natural Health for Dogs and Cats*:

"A woman brought in a cat a couple of weeks after it had been violently shaken by a large dog. The animal was uncomfortable, irritable and constipated. It had a fever, weight loss, fluid accumulation in the lungs, and a painful abdomen. The most severe injury seemed to be a displaced vertebra in the lower back ...

"I prescribed ... Star of Bethlehem, two drops to be given every two hours. Three days later, the cat's owner called to say that her cat was quite recovered."

30. Sweet Chestnut

General indications – given to encourage those who are suffering from complete and utter anguish and despair. The Sweet Chestnut state comes at the end of the road, where everything is bleak and not even death offers a way out.

This remedy is often used along with Star of Bethlehem for cats that have given up on life after the death of a beloved human or feline companion. It can also be used for very ill animals that appear to be in great anguish.

Things to look for:

♡ genuine suffering.

♡ grave or terminal illness.

♡ cats that seem to have lost all hope, where you yourself can see no solution.

♡ inconsolable grief.

31. Vervain

General indications – used to give more balance and poise to those who are overfull of life and commitment. Sometimes enthusiasm goes too far and leads to emotional and physical burnout, or to fanaticism, and Vervain is the remedy when this state of imbalance threatens.

The Vervain cat can't wait to get out and about in the morning, and greets every visitor with a display of exuberance. There seems to be a genetic pre-disposition towards Vervain in some small, thin and agile cats such as Burmese and Siamese – the kind of cats that like to dash up the curtains and along the rafters!

Things to look for:

♡ over-exuberance and over-enthusiasm.

♡ over-excitability and over-activity.

♡ fiery anger at injustice.

♡ cats that quickly get frustrated or angry when illness and incapacity mean that they cannot be about their normal affairs.

32. Vine

General indications – this remedy is used to encourage the positive side of leadership in those who sometimes use force to get their own way. Vine types know their own minds and want others to do things their way, and in a negative state don't much care how they achieve this.

The Vine cat is the true dominant, and in the wild would always be ready to test itself against possible rivals in the group. The remedy encourages a gentler side to the qualities of determination and strength, so that the cat can assert itself and assume leadership without necessarily having to use force.

Things to look for:

♡ bullying of other cats or kittens.

♡ physical threats and intimidation.

♡ insistence on being first for food, cuddles etc.

Cat psychologist Peter Neville is a particular fan of Vine, as he explains in his 1990 book *Cat Behaviour Explained*:

"Never have I encountered more success with using Bach Flower Remedies than with treating despots. Four drops of Vine, diluted with water and squirted into the cat's mouth via a plastic pipette two or three times a day, if it won't be accepted in drinking water or milk, has produced some amazing results. Despots ... are still arrogant strutters, but instead of attacking their usual victim, they simply ignore them or, at worst, hiss and walk away. I wish someone could tell me why this treatment is so effective ..."

33. Walnut

General indications – given to those who are being led astray by outside influences, past or present, and to those who are going through a time of change and need help to adjust.

Sometimes Walnut is given to cats that are having trouble being themselves because of the influence of other, more dominant cats – although Centaury (see above) may be a better choice in many cases. Otherwise, the commonest use for Walnut is when a change in the cat's universe has had an unsettling effect. Moving house, the arrival of a new cat rival in the household, guests coming to stay – all these situations suggest Walnut as a likely remedy.

Things to look for:

♡ cats that need help adjusting to changes such as moving
house or the arrival of new companions.

♡ cats struggling to cope with life changes, such as
weaning, pregnancy, disability, infirmity in old age etc.

♡ independent cats that come under the influence of
another more dominant cat or are otherwise disturbed
by neighbours, children and so on.

34. Water Violet

General indications – sometimes self-reliance and a liking for
one's own company can build up barriers to the rest of cre-
ation, leaving one isolated and unable to make contact with
others. Water Violet is the remedy to help soften those in this
state so that they can take the steps necessary to help the barriers come down.

Cats are often thought of as all being Water Violet types –
independent, aloof and preferring to be alone. In fact they are
like any other creature in that they can be Water Violets or they
can be other types – it depends on the individual. And the cat
that displays apparently aloof behaviour, such as not making
eye contact and even turning its back on someone, is actually
demonstrating anxiety and submission.

True Water Violet cats are not shy or fearful like Mimulus cats,
but simply prefer to be by themselves. The Water Violet remedy
helps when they need support but no longer know how to get it.

Things to look for:

♡ cats that are aloof and reject familiarity, but show no
sign of fear.

♡ loners that keep to themselves.

35. White Chestnut

General indications – used to still worrying, repetitive thoughts and mental arguments.

In this state cats may appear distracted, agitated or inattentive. Something in their lives is bothering them and stopping them from concentrating on what they are doing – which is why this remedy may help settle queens that are in season.

Things to look for:

♡ restlessness during sleep.

♡ insomnia.

♡ inability to concentrate or to enjoy quiet moments.

36. Wild Oat

General indications – this remedy is given to those who want to do something worthwhile with their lives but don't know what that something should be. They feel frustrated at their lack of commitment and purpose, and may drift through lack of direction.

In the case of cats this remedy state can be difficult to spot, so you are relying a lot on your intuition. Wild Oat can be useful – used along with Walnut – when an activity that was once enjoyed is now no longer possible, so that the cat is left without an aim in life. This could happen to a cat that has always lived an active outdoor life, and now through old age or incapacity is forced to live indoors, where it mopes around never settling at any activity and seeming frustrated and unsatisfied with everything. Taking Wild Oat will allow it to focus better and discover what it really enjoys doing so that it can find new purpose in life.

Things to look for:

♡ aimless behaviour.

♡ inability to settle in one particular lifestyle.

37. Wild Rose

General indications – given to those who resign themselves without struggling to whatever life throws their way. In a positive state they are happy-go-lucky and relaxed but when out of balance they feel that life is passing them by.

Cats that have been sick for a long time can fall into a Wild Rose state. They become reluctant to return to normal activities such as going outside, and the Wild Rose remedy can help to get them over the hump. (See also Hornbeam.)

Things to look for:

♡ lack of interest in life.

♡ general apathy.

♡ cats that are fit and well but lack energy and motivation.

38. Willow

General indications – used to encourage a more positive, generous outlook in those who blame others for their troubles and sink into grumbling resentment and self-pity.

Willow can be useful for cats that resent the introduction of a new kitten or puppy into the household. In these circumstances it would commonly be given in conjunction with Walnut and possibly Mimulus.

Things to look for:

♡ persistent, complaining vocal sounds – or, more likely, complete silence and lack of movement.

♡ sullen refusal to respond to friendly overtures.

Rescue Remedy (39)

Rescue Remedy is a combination of five remedies ready-mixed for emergency use. It contains:

♡ Star of Bethlehem (shock)

♡ Clematis (faintness)

♡ Rock Rose (terror and panic)

♡ Cherry Plum (loss of self-control)

♡ Impatiens (agitation and irritability)

Rescue Remedy can be thought of as a single remedy with its own indications, which is why it is sometimes referred to as the 39th remedy. It can help whenever a cat under pressure needs some help to stay calm and in control.

The Bach Centre receives countless testimonials each year from happy cat-lovers who have found Rescue Remedy useful. Here are two recent examples from friends in the USA:

♡ "I just wanted to write and say how much I love Rescue Remedy. I do volunteer animal rescue and have used it on my cats/kittens for a myriad of things. I used it on two kittens who I truly believed would have died without it."

♡ "I've had wonderful success treating my cats with Rescue Remedy. Take a feral I'm trying to tame – he was clawing, hissing, spitting and biting. I began giving him four drops in his water twice a day and four drops in a little canned cat food. Earlier this evening he let me pet him. I think that's incredible progress in just six days. I also began putting four drops in the big communal bowl of water for my other residents (there are nine, eight females and the last one, a year-old three-legged male) who were still a bit skittish about territory since the big boy moved in. There hasn't been even the threat of a disturbance yet. You have my wholehearted endorsement!"

Rescue Remedy is the remedy most often given to cats, probably because it is an obvious way of helping a cat keep calm in a difficult situation. However, it is not a panacea for all ills. Once the immediate stress has been dealt with the long-term solution lies in mixing an individual combination of remedies for your particular, individual cat. There is no danger involved in using the Rescue Remedy over a long period of time, but it will not necessarily cure deep-seated imbalances – for that you need to turn to the system of 38 remedies.

Things to look for:

♥ emergency situations that leave the cat dazed, disorientated, frightened, upset etc.

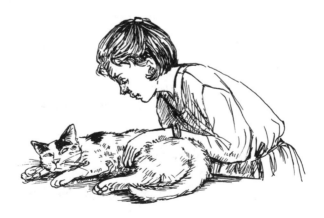

♡ any first-aid situation where there is no time to make a balanced assessment and you need help fast while you wait for the vet.

Rescue Cream

Rescue Cream is a soft, non-greasy, lanolin-free cream. It contains Rescue Remedy and Crab Apple, which is chosen for its cleansing qualities.

Rescue Cream might appear to be an exception to the rule that says that the remedies treat emotional states. This is because it is usually applied to physical problems such as skin disorders, rashes, minor cuts, bruises and so on. However, the cream is simply a convenient way of applying Rescue Remedy and Crab Apple externally, in much the same way as a practitioner might give a mix of remedies selected for an emotional state and apply the same remedies in a compress to any external manifestation of the underlying emotional disorder.

The kind of problems Rescue Cream treats are usually accompanied by some form of emotional stress or crisis (which explains the Rescue Remedy in the cream), or by a feeling of contamination and dislike of ones own appearance (which accounts for the presence of Crab Apple). Just as Rescue Remedy would be useful for someone who has fallen downstairs, so the Cream can be used to treat the external manifestation of the crisis.

Selecting remedies for cats

In one respect it is easier to help cats with Bach Flower Remedies than it is to help people. Cats do not usually carry as much emotional baggage as the average adult human. What you see is what you get. Once the correct remedies have been identified they can work quickly to resolve the situation, although cats that have suffered major psychological damage may take many months to improve. The main difficulty, then, lies in making that first selection. We can't expect cats to sit up and tell us why they are anxious. Neither can we ask them whether they doubt their own judgement, or if they are worried about something.

The typical cat response to a difficult situation is to get away from it. If flight is not possible the cat will fight, or simply freeze in place and avoid eye contact. One way or another they shut down communication with us, and they do it in ways that almost invite us to misunderstand them. Cats that look away and freeze when a child approaches, or immediately turn and walk away, may seem to the onlooker to be coldly refusing a friendly overture. In fact they are frightened or nervous of the child, and avoiding the problem as best they can. It is all too easy to misread the reason for a response like this, and so select the wrong remedy. To minimise the chance of this happening we need to try to understand what is happening from the cat's point of view.

It helps to think first about cats in general and the way they live and interact. All cats share a fundamental approach to life, just as all people are human and look at life in a human way. We can try to empathise with the feline species and get a feel for the kind of emotions that cats might feel in particular situations. For example, cats are highly evolved hunters, pre-programmed to be interested in small, fast objects, and to burn energy in the pursuit of them. They are unlikely to be happy in a dull environment with nothing to chase. They are social animals and need interaction with other cats, and failing that, time with humans. They will not thrive if they are locked in an empty apartment most of the day and will do even worse if they get no input from you when you finally arrive home from work. And because they are not pack animals, they will not be especially loyal to you or your family. They will welcome food and social interaction with the people next door just as readily as they take it from you.

Cat breeds

It can be helpful to think about what breed your cat is, because there are often clear genetic links between particular physical attributes and certain emotional outlooks. This is a bit like breaking down humanity according to ethnic type – rational, cool-headed Scandinavians on the one hand, hot-blooded, vivacious Latins on the other – and as with all such generalizations you need to take it with a very large pinch of salt. Knowing a breed's characteristics will not let you predict behaviour and personality in an individual cat, and all cats are capable of all kinds of feline behaviour – but you will at least know which types of personality and behaviour are more likely than others. Here then are basic character sketches of some of the more popular breeds, starting with the shorthairs.

Shorthairs

Most cats are shorthaired, for the simple reason that in the wild this is the most practical way to be: short hair offers no advantage to potential enemies and is easy to clean. Even pedigree shorthairs may only be a few generations away from street cats, which may explain why they tend to be more outgoing and self-reliant than longhairs. The following tendencies have been noticed in specific breeds and the questions are simply to encourage you to think about the different remedies and how they can be applied.

- ♡ Abyssinians can be easier to train than other cats – might Centaury apply more often than Chestnut Bud?

- ♡ American Shorthairs are known to be especially energetic – might Vervain be more useful than Wild Rose?

- ♡ British Blue Shorthairs sometimes avoid noise and bustle, although they are still affectionate and mischievous when they are in the mood – could Water Violet be more appropriate than Chicory?

- ♡ Burmese cats are known to have an especial affection for people – might Red Chestnut or Chicory be useful in the right circumstances?

- ♡ Exotic Shorthairs are crosses between short- and longhairs, and as such are a mix of gentleness and playfulness – would this rule out Vine as a type remedy?

- ♡ Moggies – or street cats – come in all shapes, sizes and personalities. They tend to be healthier and hardier than so-called 'pure-bred' cats – perhaps more likely to need Oak than Gentian?

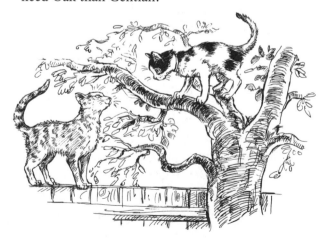

♡ Russian Blues are quiet, shy and amenable – could Centaury or Mimulus be useful here?

♡ Siamese are extrovert and boisterous; they may become so attached to their humans that they try to keep them to themselves – Vervain, perhaps, or Chicory, or even Holly when jealousy gets out of hand?

Longhairs

Longhairs are usually pedigree cats, or bred from pedigree cats, and are not 'designed' for life in the wild. Indeed many of them could not survive without the diligent care of a human, who can keep them groomed and in a healthy condition. In general they are relaxed, gentle and good-tempered. In addition to these base characteristics, breeders have noted the following tendencies in particular breeds:

♡ Balinese cats enjoy playing with their kittens and are especially fond of human company – could Chicory apply at times?

♡ Black Longhairs are livelier than most. They are affectionate with people they know but can be suspicious of new acquaintances – Holly might help unfounded suspicion, perhaps?

♡ Chinchilla Longhairs are sometimes temperamental and moody – how about Scleranthus where moods come and go rapidly, or Mustard if they seem gloomy for no apparent reason?

♡ Chocolate Longhairs may show more curiosity than most longhairs – could Vervain be a good choice for a tired Chocolate?

♡ Colourpoint Longhairs are lively and not too disruptive – how common would a Vervain state be in this breed?

♡ Lilac Longhairs are friendly and extrovert – might Heather or Agrimony apply if they are always on the lookout for company and find it hard to be alone?

♡ Norwegian Forest cats may be demanding and expect lots of attention – could they have Chicory tendencies?

♡ Ragdoll cats, as the name suggests, relax and go floppy when picked up. They are especially tolerant of clumsy humans but the idea that they do not feel pain is complete nonsense – might Agrimony describe their easy-going natures and willingness to conceal pain?

♡ Somali cats may be shy of strangers – would this mean they would need Mimulus more than Vine?

♡ Tabby Longhairs tend to show more independence – could Water Violet be a likely type remedy?

♡ Tortoiseshell Longhairs are especially noted for being good mothers – is this the good mothering of a Chicory cat, or the anxiousness of Red Chestnut, or the enthusiasm of Vervain, or the over-care of Vine?

♡ White Longhairs may be overly fussy about cleanliness and appearance – could Crab Apple help?

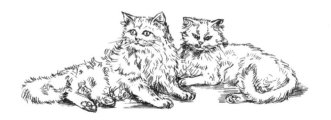

Cat personality types

Any of the 38 remedies could apply to any cat, regardless of breed. So having thought about cats in general and having gained a further insight from the breed of your cat, you need to consider its temperament. Think about the particular cat that you want to help. What tells it apart from every other cat? How would you describe its natural temperament – is it aggressive, or highly strung, or sociable, or loving, or gentle? Think about how it tends to act when things go wrong – does it go very quiet and withdraw, or protest loudly? Is it assertive and extrovert or introverted and put-upon?

The answers to these questions will guide you towards probable *type remedies* for your cat. A type remedy is a remedy that describes the cat's fundamental personality and by extension tells you how it will probably feel whenever it is out of balance, either through illness or because of life's slings and arrows.

There is no fixed list of type remedies, but the most commonly used cat type remedies are probably:

- ♡ Mimulus – shy, timid types that avoid crowds and keep out of the way of strangers.

- ♡ Impatiens – quick-thinking, impetuous types that are always in a hurry and get irritable if they are held up.

- ♡ Vine – boss cats who use threats and aggression to assert themselves.

- ♡ Chicory – cats that love to be the centre of the family's attention and find it difficult to give freedom to loved humans, kittens or feline friends.

- ♡ Beech – can't understand why other cats or people don't do the same as them, and are intolerant of different approaches, new things etc.

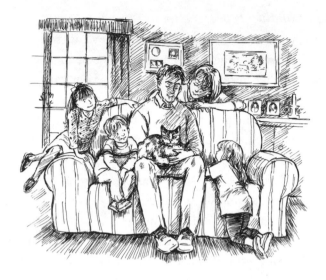

♡ Vervain – enthusiastic cats that throw themselves into their favourite pursuits without considering the cost.

♡ Centaury – born followers and helpers, they may be dominated by others and lose their independence.

♡ Heather – displaying self-absorption without self-respect, Heather cats crave attention from anyone.

♡ Scleranthus – eternal ditherers, going from one thing to another without making up their minds either way.

♡ Clematis – excessively dreamy, sleepy types that seem to need more than the average cat's sixteen hours of rest a day.

♡ Wild Rose – easy-going drifters that don't often get enthusiastic about life or anything in it.

♡ Water Violet – cats that are especially happy with their own company and avoid spending time with all but a couple of select individuals.

♡ Agrimony – cats that play the fool even when they are in pain or suffering.

♡ Larch – cats that avoid challenges and don't try to cope with difficulties.

♡ Oak – strong, slow, dependable, deliberate cats that do not know when they are beaten.

♡ Crab Apple – fussy, obsessive cats.

♡ Rock Water – the ascetics of the cat world, they avoid rest in order to keep to their routine.

As with all remedy descriptions, these stress the negative, since it is in the negative state that the remedies are needed. But each type has a positive, balanced aspect as well. A positive Vine is a wise leader, a positive Heather a great companion and sharer of sorrows, a positive Beech a tolerant, understanding neighbour.

Cat moods

Having thought about her personality, ask yourself how your cat seems right now. Is she particularly sleepy, hyperactive, aggressive, frightened or lethargic? Does she seem to be afraid of something, or look like she has had a shock, or does she have no energy, or want to be petted, or to be left alone? And have you noticed anything in particular that seems to be associated with this behaviour? Has a stranger just come to visit the house? Is this the first time your cat has seen a man with a beard? Or does she always get over-excited or anxious when a particular voice comes on the radio or when you visit certain places, or at the sight of her food bowl or scratching post?

Questions like these will guide you to the *mood remedies* your cat needs. A mood remedy is simply a remedy that matches the way your cat feels at the moment. So while an Impatiens type cat will tend to get irritable whenever there is a delay, any cat can be in an Impatiens state given the right circumstances. One might need Impatiens at feeding time, while another will only need it when the children stop her from going to sleep when she wants to.

All of the 38 remedies can be mood remedies.

The art of choosing a remedy

Selecting remedies involves using your powers of observation, calling on your own knowledge of cats in general and of your cat in particular, plus a good dose of gut feeling, intuition and common sense, in order to determine as far as you can your cat's current state of mind. Once you think you know how she feels and why she is acting the way she is, simply select the remedies that match.

Try not to over-analyse. Keep it simple and treat what you see. If your cat does not need one of the remedies you give her then that remedy will have no effect. Even if you select all the wrong remedies at least you know you will not make things worse.

Giving remedies to cats

There is no danger of your cat overdosing on remedies. She needs to take enough remedy, but it does not matter if she takes more than she needs. With this in mind, the dosage instructions here are for the minimum dose.

Basically, dosage for cats is the same as for humans: 4 drops of Rescue Remedy and/or 2 drops of any of the 38 remedies, diluted in a 30ml (1oz) bottle of water. Use mineral water for preference, as this keeps fresh for longer. You can mix from one to seven remedies together at a time. If you include Rescue Remedy in a mix it counts as one remedy. Give 4 drops from the mixed treatment bottle at a time, by mouth, at regular intervals, four times a day. You can give more frequent doses if you want, and doing so can be a good way of getting through a crisis.

You can give the remedies in less dilute form, or even neat if it is more convenient, although be aware that the effects are no stronger and some cats do not like the taste or smell of the brandy in the stock bottle. For example, you could fill your cat's drinking vessel with fresh water and add 4 drops of Rescue Remedy. Your cat will then get a dose of Rescue Remedy each time it drinks. You can do the same with one or a combination of the 38 individual remedies as well – the dosage being 2 drops of each one. Just add a further dose of the remedies each time you change the water.

The problem with this approach is that many cats hardly seem to drink at all. They get all the water they need from their food. If your cat does not drink regularly try adding remedies to its food as well, or giving them via a small biscuit or piece of bread offered four times a day. You may need to be more imaginative if your cat is off its food altogether. You could drip the remedy around his lips, or onto the ears or feet – cats will quickly lick the liquid off and get the remedies that way.

The idea is to make it convenient for you to give the remedies, and easy and unstressful for your cat to take them. You can use any method that you want, as long as your cat gets at least the minimum dose of 4 drops from a treatment bottle, four times a day.

Treating yourself

It is easy to get so wrapped up in choosing remedies for your cat that you forget to think about your own needs. A distressed cat means a distressed family because when any loved animal is ill or is simply not itself its owners will be emotionally involved. Don't forget to use the remedies to help everyone in the family stay on top of their emotions. Any of the 38 remedies may apply, and the following are just some of many possible examples:

- ♡ Red Chestnut for anxiety about the animal's welfare.

- ♡ Star of Bethlehem for shock, either after an accident or when a serious illness has been diagnosed.

- ♡ Gentian for despondency; or Gorse if you feel very pessimistic.

- ♡ White Chestnut for constant worry.

- ♡ Agrimony if you try to put a brave face on things but feel upset underneath.

- ♡ Vervain for anger and frustration at the injustice of it all; or Willow if your anger is laced with self-pity.

- ♡ Impatiens if you simply feel irritated by what is happening, and want the problem to go away at once.

- ♡ Pine if you blame yourself for some act or omission that has caused the problem or made it worse.

Some people will find the illness of an animal harder to cope with than others. Children, the elderly, and those who live alone can be hit particularly hard, especially when the animal does not recover and eventually dies. In these circumstances too the remedies can be helpful:

- ♡ Star of Bethlehem for shock and for the sense of grief and loss.

- ♡ Sweet Chestnut when it feels that there is nothing left to live for and that the feeling will never go away.

- ♡ Walnut to help adjust to the new circumstances.

♡ Honeysuckle to help bring the mind away from the past and back into the present (this can be especially helpful for older people who have lost a companion).

Your cat will benefit if you take the time to help yourself and the rest of your family with the remedies, whatever the eventual outcome of any illness. You will be able to think clearly and be more objective about selecting remedies for your cat if you are in control of your own emotions. More importantly, your cat's own emotional state will be better if you and your family are in balance. Just as an animal's distress can trigger distress within the family so the reverse is true, and a distressed family can be distressing for an animal. Your cat is a sensitive creature that is likely to be affected by any severe or prolonged negative emotion you may be experiencing. In response she may display symptoms of stress – anxiety, depression, guilt, fear, worry – as though empathising with your own feelings. People who work with animals have long recognised that emotions like anxiety are infectious. The old joke that people and their pets come to look like each other may not be true, but they certainly tend to share each other's neuroses. Indeed, you may find yourself looking for remedies to help your cat when in fact your cat's emotional state is simply a manifestation of your own. Bearing in mind one of the most important principles of Dr Bach's work – treat the cause, not the effect – the remedies you want to give to your cat may be the remedies that you should be taking yourself.

The principle of treating yourself first applies in particular to situations where there is no actual illness, but rather an apparent behavioural or emotional problem such as separation anxiety. You may go out of your way to make a huge fuss of your cat every time you come home. You have to be out most of the time, but you want him to know that you love him and care for him. Then you are surprised when he starts mewing and trying to stop you from leaving the house again, and think that he probably needs Chicory because he is so clingy. Take Chicory yourself before giving it to your cat, because you are the one who is creating his emotional dependency by deliberately setting out to win his love.

Our unreasonable expectations and misreading of situations often lead us to see the cat as a problem where in fact the problem is us. Compared with the aeons they spent living wild, cats have been domesticated for a very short time. They still think and live more like hunters than pampered pets. If we keep a cat shut up alone in a tiny flat it will suffer, either visibly (holes in the curtains and urine on the carpet) or in secret (quiet desperation under the sofa). Vervain or Mimulus or Willow or Gorse will help to an extent, but the real cure lies in our attitude towards a fellow creature. If we are going to invite cats into our houses it must be at least partly on their terms, and not wholly on ours.

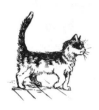

Part Two

Treating feline emotions

Bach Flower Remedies do not treat physical complaints directly. They can't get rid of a fur ball trapped in your cat's gut or mend her broken leg – although they can help her feel less sorry for herself while the leg gets better. Where a disease is stress-related Bach Flower Remedies will treat the underlying emotional cause, but separate treatment may be needed to deal with the symptomatic disease. You should always consider other methods of treatment as a complement to the remedies for any physical illness or condition.

First aid

Injuries
Injuries to cats are usually the result of human carelessness and feline curiosity. Cats fall from open windows, are cut by can lids and broken bottles and get their tails shut in doors. Other injuries are the result of bites – and for obvious reasons entire toms are especially at risk. A bite from another cat can be dangerous, and if there is infection it is liable to be out of sight and deep inside the wound. Applying an antiseptic will not necessarily do any good and you should consult a vet.

♡ In all cases of injury reach for Rescue Remedy. For minor wounds where the cat will recover by itself this will help it calm down and not be distressed by the event. Where the injury is more serious it will help while you seek veterinary attention. (And take it yourself at the same time.)

♡ Apply Rescue Cream to minor wounds and scratches – with open wounds, however, get veterinary advice before applying anything.

♡ If there is severe and uncontrollable bleeding press down on the wound with a pad of some kind (anything will do in an emergency – from a wad of cotton wool to a tee-shirt). Give Rescue Remedy by mouth, or apply it to lips, gums and ears.

♡ Do not remove objects such as nails and glass from a wound, since this may make things worse. Instead roll up a piece of cloth into a ring and place it around the object, then bandage the pad in place.

♡ In severe cases cover the cat with a sweater, blanket or even a piece of kitchen foil – this will keep its body temperature up while you wait for help to arrive.

Stings

Cats will stalk anything that moves. This means they are likely to get stung from time to time, especially in the cool of spring and summer, when bees and wasps are drowsy and easier to catch. Kittens are especially at risk because they have not learned to avoid stripy insects.

♡ Bathe sore, red areas around a sting with cold water and Rescue Remedy.

♡ Give Rescue Remedy by mouth to calm a frightened or distressed cat.

Travel and travel sickness

Cats can be good travellers, but they need time to get used to the idea. That means taking a few short trips in the car before you attempt the 100-mile trip to a new home. It also means that if your cat cannot stand getting into the car you will have to spend some time getting it used to the idea. You could try feeding it in the parked car for a few days, to get it used to the smell, then gradually work up to a short drive a few yards up the road. As with all retraining, the key is to build up slowly and go back to the previous stage if there is any kind of setback.

Travel-sick cats tend to vomit and may salivate profusely. They will find motion less upsetting if they are carried in a securely fastened basket kept (if possible) down near the floor. Some owners find that a few reminders of home also help, such as a favourite blanket or toy. They reduce anxiety – and a few toys will also give your cat something to do while travelling.

The following remedies can be used to help cats cope with motion sickness and with travel anxieties in general:

♡ Scleranthus has been found to be useful for travel sickness.

♡ Mimulus will help deal with any specific anxieties to do with getting into the car, or being put into a travelling basket etc.

♡ Where a cat loses control completely and panics or works itself into a frenzy, consider Rock Rose or Cherry Plum, or give Rescue Remedy, which contains both.

♡ Walnut can be helpful for cats that are upset by changes.

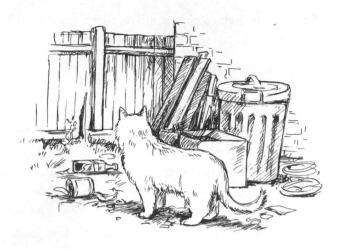

♡ Try Chestnut Bud if you are having to retrain a cat to accept occasional journeys, and find it is particularly slow to learn.

Burns

Cats do not get burned very often, and when they do it is normally the result of human carelessness. Number one cause is probably spilt tea, coffee and boiling water – but burns can also come from electrical and chemical sources.

Oil, butter and Rescue Cream should never be applied to burns at the time they happen. The heat in the burn would fry the oil or cream and cause more damage. Instead cool the affected area by applying a liquid that will evaporate the heat and cool down the skin. Cold water is the best thing for this, and the sooner you use it the better. Add Rescue Remedy to the water to help soothe the trauma. If there is no water to hand you can drip neat Rescue Remedy onto the burn and it will have the same effect. Give Rescue Remedy by mouth (or rub it on gums) at the same time, so as to help your cat recover the sooner from the stress.

If the burn is anything more than very minor seek the assistance of your veterinary surgeon as soon as possible.

Heatstroke

The old and the young are most at risk from heatstroke, but obese cats are also especially prone to this problem, as are long-haired cats in general. Cats with heatstroke tend to pant to try to lose the excess heat, and they can lose consciousness.

If your cat suffers anything more than mild heatstroke you should seek veterinary advice at once. In the meantime the essential thing is to cool the cat down as quickly as possible. Cold water is the quickest solution – immerse the cat's body in it, keeping the head up so that it can breathe, or if this is not possible then wet the cat thoroughly. A bag of frozen vegetables from the freezer makes a quick and effective ice pack, and you should offer drinks to help reduce heat and avoid dehydration.

♡ Give Rescue Remedy or Star of Bethlehem at frequent intervals. The same remedies can be added to cold water and drinks or dropped onto ears, rubbed onto gums and so on.

Choking

Occasionally cats try to swallow something they shouldn't. In most cases the cat can clear the obstruction by itself – but occasionally it needs a little help.

♡ Give Rescue Remedy to keep the cat calm – and take it yourself.

♡ Try to remove the obstruction with your fingers.

♡ Where it is not possible to remove the obstruction seek immediate veterinary help.

♡ If the cat cannot breathe at all, vet Roger Taylor (*The Ultimate Cat Book*) recommends picking up the cat by the hind legs and vigorously swinging it around so that centrifugal force will expel the obstruction.

Emotion and behaviour

Aggression

You might be familiar with the way a cat will rough-house quite happily with your hand, but then as soon as you roll it over onto its back it will attack you and rake your forearm or hand with its back claws. This is fear-based aggression – you are paying the price of putting the cat into a vulnerable position where it feels anxious.

Fear is the most likely cause of aggression towards human beings. Where there is aggression towards other cats, however,

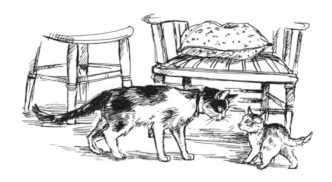

there might be other reasons such as the need to establish dominance or defend territory from an intruder. You will see aggression like this when a new cat moves into a house where an existing cat is already living. It can be reduced if the two cats are introduced gradually. Try keeping the new cat shut in a room by itself for a few days, so as to give the older tenant a chance to get used to the idea that there is a new friend in town.

Different types of aggression need different remedies, so you will need to give some thought as to why your cat feels aggressive. You might get it wrong a few times before you hit on the right explanation. There is no problem with selecting remedies by trial and error because they can't do any harm. Here are some examples of remedies that might apply:

♡ Mimulus where the cat lashes out through fear, and you can identify a reason for the fear. Look for attacks on particular individuals (children, the man next door, your husband) or in particular situations (at the vet's, whenever a stranger approaches) as these indicate that the cat may be afraid of something specific.

♡ Cherry Plum where the cat seems to lose its self-control and attacks whoever is nearest it, even without apparent provocation.

♡ Vine where the cat is attacking another cat and you feel that it is trying to assert its dominance. Look for particular triggers. Perhaps the attacks only happen when a favourite spot is taken by its rival, or when you make a fuss of the other cat. (In the latter case you might also try Holly to deal with the jealousy.)

♡ Beech where the cat cannot seem to tolerate the presence of the other cat at all, and always lashes out when it is there.

♡ Try Impatiens for flashes of temper that go as quickly as they come, especially if the trigger is a delay of some kind, such as not providing food at the normal hour or taking too much time to open the door.

♡ Vervain where the aggressor joins in to defend a weaker victim, but gets carried away and goes too far.

♡ Walnut where the aggression follows a change of some sort, such as the arrival of a new cat (or baby) in the house.

♡ Red Chestnut or Chicory where aggression is shown by a mother cat towards cats and people who get too close to the babies. Red Chestnut is a fear remedy, and is appropriate where fear for the safety of the kittens accounts for aggressive behaviour. With Chicory there is no fear, only a desire to stop others from enjoying the attentions of the kittens.

♡ Water Violet may be appropriate for cats that really do prefer to be alone, and lash out as a last resort when faced with insistent cat lovers – but consider Mimulus first. Other last resort aggressors would include Centaury cats, which do anything to avoid trouble and satisfy demands made on them.

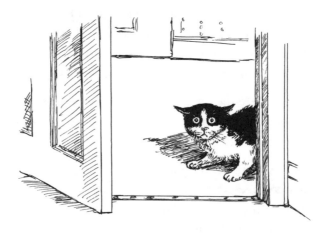

Anxiety

Cats that seem depressed or aggressive or upset are often in a state of fear. This is especially true in human/feline relationships. The difference in size and power means that any cat that is unsure of our intentions is likely to feel afraid.

Fears can go back to kittenhood and beyond. Some cat breeders don't handle kittens at an early enough age, and as grown-ups those cats will rarely be entirely at ease with people. Other cats inherit anxiety in the same way they inherit eye colour and length of fur. But other fears are contingent and, by definition, last less time and are easier to resolve. Typical examples would include nervous reactions to the noise of fireworks, and the cat that shies away from children because a child once pulled its tail. Medical treatment can cause fear. Surgery can be a daunting prospect, and cats often seem to know that something is going on. The remedies are an enormous help in relieving any apprehension, so that your cat feels calmer and less afraid. More centred in itself, it will make a quicker and fuller recovery.

Finally, fear is by far the commonest cause of feline aggression towards humans. Even the most reserved and mild of cats will eventually attack if it is frightened enough – and what to us is a simple game can easily appear to a cat as a threat to life and limb.

The fearful, anxious cat is easy to spot. It will keep low to the ground and creep around, hide behind furniture or under the bed, or just hunch up and try to ignore everything around it. It will hold its tail low and its pupils will be dilated. Whenever you spot anxiety and fear you should consider the following remedies:

♡ Mimulus if the anxiety has a definite cause that you and
   the cat can identify, such as dogs or strangers or going
   to the vet. Where possible take steps to habituate the cat

to the fearful thing. Mimulus also applies if the cat seems to be a shy and nervous type in general.

♡ Aspen if there is no apparent reason for the fear. Cats in an Aspen state will run and hide as if there were some threat around, when in fact no threat can be seen.

♡ Red Chestnut where you feel that the cat is overly-anxious either about you or about its kittens or cat friends. The Red Chestnut fear is altruistic. The cat sits in the window watching for your return and only relaxes when you are home again. Unlike a Chicory cat, however, it will not be especially attentive when it knows for a fact that you are home safe.

♡ Cherry Plum for the kind of fear that leads to loss of control and irrational and sometimes violent acts. A cat in this state will lose its ability to control its actions, and may strike out at you as you try to help it, or injure itself in its desire to escape a perceived threat.

♡ Rock Rose for absolute terror. A cat in a Rock Rose state may be so frightened of something that it is unable to act at all, or it may run away without attempting to deal with the cause of the fear.

Behavioural changes

When a cat suddenly starts to behave differently or in unexpected ways take it to a vet. Organic illnesses can cause a change in behaviour, and some of them such as encephalitis and meningitis, are serious. A cat that suddenly starts to avoid you could have been run over or suffered a fall, and one that starts to overeat is as likely to be suffering from worms as from stress. If you take your cat to the vet for a check up when it starts to behave unusually, then you will be able to nip any physical problem in the bud with luck before it becomes too serious.

You can also start to use the remedies straight away. Here are some examples of remedies that could apply to certain types of behavioural change:

♡ Give Scleranthus when there are sudden shifts of mood, from euphoria to melancholy and back again, or when the cat seems never to settle at an even keel.

♡ Select Aspen when your cat becomes fearful for no apparent reason, or suddenly starts to behave anxiously in normal everyday situations.

♡ Consider Crab Apple for cats that seem reluctant to eat their normal food, and for cats that are distressed by incontinence.

♡ Try Mustard when your cat seems morose and depressed for no reason.

♡ Try Hornbeam if your normally lively cat seems to lack the energy to enjoy life. (Consider Wild Rose and Olive as well.)

♡ Choose Walnut if you can trace the change in behaviour to a change in the cat's life, such as the arrival of new neighbours or a new cat in the family.

Depression

Depression in cats has many causes, just as in humans. Some are physical, such as suffering from illness. Others are purely mental – missing an absent friend, for example. And some are a mix of the two, such as the queen that has suffered an abortion due to an infection. Prolonged depression, as with all behavioural changes, is a sign that the cat should see a vet for a check up to ensure there is no organic cause.

Whatever the cause of the problem, there are a number of remedies that can help. Here are some of the most likely:

♡ Gentian where the cat seems a little despondent due to something going wrong – for example not getting a favourite titbit, or feeling unwell, or someone refusing to play – and just needs a little encouragement.

♡ Gorse where the cat seems to have given up and adopted a pessimistic attitude. There seems no hope, even though there might be possible solutions to hand.

♡ Mustard where there seems no reason for the cat's unhappiness.

♡ Willow where the cat seems resentful and is uncharacteristically silent. Willow cats feel sorry for themselves and seem to be sulking.

♡ Where there is serious illness or the cat is near death and suffering extreme anguish, then Sweet Chestnut may bring some relief.

Feeding problems

Imagine the following scenario. You are trying to give your cat a new food. It sniffs at the bowl, scratches around it a little, then stalks away. Guilt-stricken, you take away the offending food and replace it with the old favourite. At once pussy returns and eats the food.

You may think – perhaps with pride – that your cat is especially dainty in its habits and will not touch the new food. You may think it is offended by your attempt to get it to change its habits. But what is really happening is that the cat is not very hungry. The scratching around is an echo of life in the wild, where cats cover over a kill so as to come back to it later. When you put out a bowl of the favourite food its especially attractive odour overrides lack of hunger, which is why the cat comes back and eats up.

Unless they are very ill, in which case they should be under the care of a vet, cats do not starve themselves to death. But they are quick learners and opportunists. They soon learn that if they do not eat the first food they are offered, then their doting owner will replace it with something else – usually their favourite food. Finicky cats are like toddlers who learn to

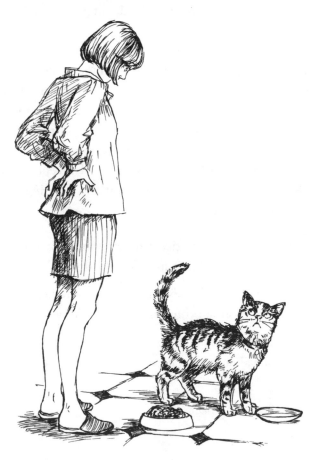

refuse mashed potato so as to hurry up the ice cream and chocolate biscuits.

Unfortunately cats do not always know best. They can become addicted to foods like liver and shellfish, and if you allow them to get away with eating nothing else their health will suffer. Even the better proprietary 'complete' foods may contain various additives and be made of fairly unwholesome ingredients. The best diet is one that mimics what cats eat in the wild – so think about the contents of the average mouse, which will include muscle, fur, innards, and the vegetable matter in the mouse's stomach. In other words, a variety of foodstuffs. By all means use a commercial cat food, but give other foods as well.

Perseverance is the key. Given time and no alternative cats will eat just about anything, and they will be healthier if you insist on a little variety. If you are having real problems feeding your cat you could try putting it on a fast for a day or two. Far from being dangerous or cruel, fasting is good for the health of already healthy cats, and mimics what would happen in the wild. After fasting even the fussiest cat will accept different foods. Remember however that pregnant and lactating queens should never be denied food.

♡ Some cats that are particularly set in their ways and intolerant of new foods may be helped with Beech.

♡ If you find it hard to say 'no' to your cat take some Centaury to stiffen your resolve at mealtimes.

♡ Red Chestnut will help you if you are worried that your cat will be hungry and upset if you try to change its diet.

(See also 'Obesity' on page 96.)

Grief

Perhaps the best-known example of grieving animals is the elephant. Elephants silently caress the bones of dead herd members, all the while remaining especially still, so that it is hard to avoid the conclusion that they are paying their last respects. Certainly, people who work closely with animals have no doubt that they feel grief and understand death. The evidence for this is so strong that even those who deny every other emotion in other animals will accept that they mourn.

Cats also miss their friends when they are no longer there. They can take up to a year to recover from the death of a companion. Along the way they display all the familiar signs, including loss of appetite and an inability to settle to ordinary tasks. Some recent studies have shown that older cats are more likely to develop life-threatening illnesses after suffering a bereavement.

Grief can also be brought about by temporary absences that may appear final to the cat. While dogs are more famous for this behaviour, cats too can suffer from the pang of separation and pine for absent friends and old familiar places.

The following remedies may help cats suffering grief:

♡ Star of Bethlehem for the shock of separation and loss. This is an ingredient in Rescue Remedy, which is also a good standby where separation has been sudden.

♡ Walnut to help adjust to the change in surroundings or companionship. Where the cat is not trying to adjust at all and is intent only on the past, then Honeysuckle would be preferred.

♡ Sweet Chestnut where a separation leads to hopelessness and complete despair. This would be the cat that really is pining away.

♥ Mimulus for cats that react to loss by displaying fear. Where the anxiety seems to be based on concern for the missing companion substitute Red Chestnut.

♥ Restless, unsettled behaviour, where the cat looks lost and unsure of itself might be helped with a number of different remedies. Start by considering Scleranthus, Cerato, Walnut, Larch and Mimulus.

We should point out that the loss of a companion, especially another cat, is not always the occasion for grief. Cats that have been bullied and pushed about by a more dominant animal can see the death of their tormentor as a blessed relief, and experience a new lease of life. However much we might deplore their innocent lack of compassion, this state does not need treatment with the remedies.

Hyperactivity

The cat's bodyclock is set differently from ours. Cats may seem hyperactive when in fact they are just playing at times that we find inconvenient. The solution will sound familiar to parents of young children – give plenty of opportunities for play at times that suit you. Then you will be more likely to get peace and quiet when you want it.

True hyperactivity is a different matter. It is characterised by insomnia and extreme alertness and activity. It may be associated with aggressive behaviour, or the cat may repeat the same action obsessively, such as continually chasing its own tail. Sometimes hyperactivity is chronic, sometimes it only emerges when the cat is under stress for some reason.

Allergies can cause hyperactivity, and additives in proprietary cat foods are often to blame. Different manufacturers use different additives, so your cat may react badly to one or two particular brands and not to others. It is worth ringing the changes every so often, and buying food from a different maker so that you can note any changes in behaviour that seem to result, and remove obvious culprits from the shopping list. Alternatively – and if you can afford to – go for the more expensive additive-free foods that are made of real meat.

♡ Where stress is causing hyperactivity, define the stress and select the appropriate remedies. Common remedies for stress include Mimulus to deal with fear and anxiety, White Chestnut for worrying thoughts, and Walnut to help adjust to changes in or around the home.

♡ Cats that are simply over-enthusiastic about the things they like and never switch off can be helped with Vervain. Another possibility is Impatiens – these cats will rush from one thing to another and get bored quickly.

♡ Crab Apple is the remedy for obsessive, repetitive behaviour.

♡ Cherry Plum may help where over-active cats relieve their frustration by grooming to the point of self-injury. Impatiens (for agitation) or Vervain (for frustration) may also help.

Spraying

A spraying cat will stand with its tail erect and its backside facing the target and squirt urine against the surface it wants to mark. Often the tail will shudder as the urine is released. Furniture, car wheels and trees are common targets, but anything can be sprayed, including your legs and those of your visitors.

Like urination, spraying is used as a way of marking out territory, but it is associated with dominance rather than fear.

Spraying cats are confident. They spray at nose height on vertical surfaces so as to be in the face of any rivals. They do not hesitate to perform the ceremony in front of other cats and outraged humans. As with the ostentatious display of faeces, spraying usually takes place around entry and exit points and in main passageways.

Spraying is most associated with entire male cats. Female cats spray as well, although they do it less often and to less effect. Neutered cats may continue to spray, although if they do it will be less often and less noticeable. Consequently vets often recommend neutering as a way of controlling the spraying of toms.

Changes in the cat's environment, stress and a local female being in heat can all trigger spraying. Remedies for the problem include not having too many cats living together, putting kitchen foil on any favourite target areas (cats don't like the noise of urine on foil), and making sure that cats have their own private bolt holes so that they do not feel the need to compete so much for territory. In addition the following remedies have been found especially useful:

♡ Walnut to help your cat adjust to unavoidable changes.

♡ Vine or Beech or Chicory to help dominant or possessive cats feel more relaxed about asserting themselves.

♡ Rescue Remedy for cats that seem to be under acute stress for some reason. This will help in the short term while you try to find the underlying reason for the spraying. Once you know the reason you can select specific remedies for your cat's individual emotional state.

Stropping

Stropping is what cats do when they reach up and claw down a tree – or all down the front arm of your new armchair. Cats use stropping to mark out territory. Other cats can see the claw marks and smell the scent left behind by glands on the stropper's paws, and know that the area has been claimed by another cat. The stropper is also reassured when it gets home and sees and smells signs of its ownership. Stropping may also be a form of isometric exercise for the cat, and of course it

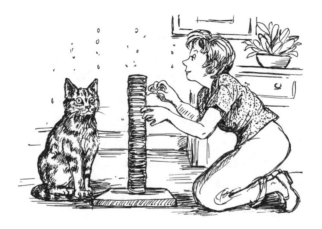

helps to keep claws sharp and ready for the hunt. With all these good reasons for stropping, your love of fine furniture is likely to be overlooked. So how do you impress on your cat that stropping is not allowed in the house?

The worst thing you can do is shout and get angry. This will only scare your cat. Instead, say a firm 'no' as soon as the cat starts to strop, and move it straight away to a proper scratching post that it *is* allowed to use. You can buy these or make them at home from wood and an old piece of carpet. If the cat persists in scratching at a particular piece of furniture place the post in front of it.

Cats are especially likely to strop new furniture. Their sensitive noses can pick up all the strange odours on the new armchair – chemicals, truck smells and the odour of the men who delivered it. This is unsettling, and by marking the new arrival they are trying to assimilate it into the den. You can help by rubbing your hands all over the new item so as to cover it with your smell. This will make it less threatening. By marking it yourself you have saved the cat a job.

♡ Walnut will help the cat adjust to changes and new arrivals.

♡ Cats that are especially intolerant of new things may need Beech. Those that are nervous will also strop threatening objects – try Mimulus or Aspen for this.

♡ Cats that fail to learn what the official scratching post is for could benefit from Chestnut Bud. And you could also consider going down on your knees in front of the scratching post and showing the cat what to do. This really does work!

Urination and soiling

Next to spraying (see above), inappropriate toilet habits are probably the commonest complaint that cat owners have about their animals. In some cases there is a physical cause, such as old age or cystitis, and for this reason any change in toilet habits or difficulty when passing water or defecating should be referred in the first instance to the vet. This is particularly important as some of the physical causes for not using litter trays can be fatal – feline urological syndrome is one and this can kill within hours.

Fortunately this sort of problem is not usually fatal, although it remains unpleasant. Some cases are down to the individual personality of your cat. Some felines are extremely fastidious and will refuse to use a litter tray if it contains the sight or smell of a previous offering. If they can't get outside they will do the next best thing and find a clean, quiet corner of your house. Longhaired cats are particularly wary of soiled trays because of the difficulty they have keeping themselves clean. The answer is as simple as making sure the litter tray is changed more frequently.

In the wild, cats will usually bury their faeces. When they do not do this, and leave them on display, it is as a visual and olfactory sign that they are claiming ownership of territory. This is why desperate gardeners have been known to borrow a bucket of lion droppings to put the fear of God into neighbourhood moggies. Dominant cats may feel the need to mark their territory in this striking way after stress-inducing behaviour on the part of feline neighbours.

Stress – and in particular fear – is a major factor in many cases of inappropriate urination. Look for any changes in your cat's routine or lifestyle, such as neighbours coming or going, a new cat, or children being born or leaving home. By leaving wet patches around the house the cat is masking the area with a familiar smell and trying to make it 'safe' again. The key difference between fear-based urination and physical incontinence is that the fearful cat will still use its litter tray to relieve its full bladder – a quick squirt of urine is all that is needed to mark an area. Urine marking is a secretive, fearful act, and you may never catch the cat in the act. Even if you do there is no point in frightening your animal still more by reprimanding it. All that will do is make the problem worse.

Finally, soiling can be caused by an allergic reaction. Have you changed the disinfectant you use on the cat's litter tray, or switched food brands, or cleaned the carpet recently? Cats can be allergic to chemicals from a wide range of sources, and soiling is one possible response.

Whatever the cause of the problem Bach Flower Remedies can be used to help.

- ♡ Where you think a change is the root of the problem, give Walnut plus specific remedies for the way your cat is reacting to the change.

- ♡ Stress caused by fear will be helped with Mimulus or Rock Rose – or use Rescue Remedy to get your cat over a crisis.

- ♡ If you feel soiling is your cat's way of claiming territory likely remedies include Chicory, Vervain and Vine.

- ♡ Especially fastidious cats that dislike sharing litter trays or refuse to use a change of litter more than one or two times could benefit from Crab Apple.

- ♡ Mimulus or Crab Apple may help cats that get distressed when they urinate inappropriately.

- ♡ Cats that always look for a private corner in which to do their business could benefit from Water Violet or Mimulus, depending on whether or not their need for privacy is related to self-reliance or shyness.

Life experiences

Being born

Cats are good mothers, and newborn kittens are small enough to emerge easily. This means that birth and the first few days of life are relatively trauma-free for most kittens. Immediately after birth the mother will clean them carefully with her tongue, digesting the birth sac and any other mess, including faeces, so as to keep the nest clean. She cuts the umbilical cord with her teeth, and the suckling kittens get a natural medicine called colostrum followed by a rich milk. This will be all that most of them need – but if necessary the remedies can provide further help in a gentle and natural way.

- ♡ Walnut to help adjust to the new world, plus Star of Bethlehem if the birth has been especially traumatic. These two remedies are commonly given at birth to human and feline new-borns alike.
- ♡ Olive if labour has been unusually prolonged and the new kitten appears weak and exhausted.
- ♡ Hornbeam where the kitten has had an easy birth but still seems slow to move.
- ♡ Clematis for kittens that seem barely alive.
- ♡ Wild Rose for kittens that make no effort to seek out their mother.
- ♡ Impatiens for kittens that seem unusually agitated.

Some breeders maintain that you can tell a lot about the personality of a kitten even before it is born. Kittens that move around a lot in the womb, and kick out strongly, will be more assertive and demanding – Vine, Impatiens, Vervain, Beech etc. Quieter kittens will turn out to be easy-going or retiring – Wild Rose, Agrimony, Centaury, Mimulus and so on.

Kittenhood

Kittens take about six months to grow up. Throughout this period they learn through play, and by imitating each other and their mother. Sometimes play among litter-mates becomes quite boisterous, and can involve lots of cuffing and biting. Injuries rarely result from this kind of activity, and for young cats it is an essential part of growing up – if anyone needs remedies it is the over-anxious owner, who should be taking Red Chestnut. We can understand the importance of play by comparing normal kittens to less fortunate animals that have been separated from their litter-mates too early, denying them the opportunity to learn in those crucial first few weeks. They tend to be more anxious, antisocial and neurotic than the average.

Kittens should not be separated from their mothers until they are at least six weeks old, and if possible they should stay with their families until they are at least eight weeks old and fully weaned. However, they *should* be handled by careful owners as early as possible, almost from birth, and every day. Handling young kittens acclimatises them to people, and makes for more intelligent, affectionate and confident cats.

As for remedies, the following are often used during the first six months of a cat's life:

♡ Mimulus for fearful kittens, and for shy, timid cats that tend to get pushed around by litter-mates. Consider Centaury and Larch as well.

♡ Walnut to help adjust to teething and weaning.

♡ Star of Bethlehem for anything that seems to come as a shock to the kitten. This could include going to a new home and being frightened by roughhousing children.

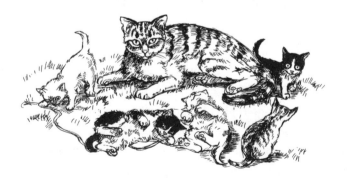

♡ Chestnut Bud for kittens that seem to take an especially long time learning to use a litter tray or a cat-flap.

♡ Rescue Remedy to get through any emergency in a calm frame of mind.

Spare a thought for the new kitten that has just left its feline family for life with a new human family. It will be disorientated and confused – where are its litter-mates and mother, and where are all its familiar cosy corners and toys? No wonder, then, that many kittens behave entirely out of character in the first week or so in a new home. Normally adventurous cats become introverted and anxious, while shy retiring types reveal unsuspected depths of aggression and activity.

Keep patient and things will settle down. If there are young children in the house, try to keep them relaxed and stop them crowding and scaring the new arrival. Wait for the kitten to make the first move to initiate a friendship. And use Walnut to help your new kitten adjust to its new environment. Try Star of Bethlehem for cats that seem particularly bereft now that mum and brothers and sisters are no longer around.

Cats and other cats

In the wild cats use scent markings left by spraying and stropping to stake out territory and avoid conflict with other cats. A cat coming across a marking will sniff at the scent, and carry on and use the territory for hunting if the mark is a few hours old. When the scent is fresh the cat will consider carefully before going on, and may in fact change course. Thanks to this system several cats can patrol the same territory without having to meet at all.

Is it true then that cats are antisocial creatures? The short answer is, no. The loner cat is largely a myth, and more cats are given Water Violet to no good purpose than any other remedy.

A number of research programmes in the 1970s showed that in a feral state domestic cats choose to live together in social groupings that resemble those adopted by their larger relatives. Like prides of lions, cats congregate around food sources. Males fight – when necessary – to establish who is dominant in the group, but often there is no need to fight since cats that are likely to lose a fight are usually sensible enough to give way. Males range more widely than females. Their territory can be ten times as wide as a female's, which allows them to patrol a number of potential mates. Where the researchers found differences between the behaviour of domestic cats and big cats these seemed to be based on food supply. Female ranges in the city-dwelling feral cat overlap because there is more food available. Female tigers and jaguars need to be jealous of their personal ranges so as to safeguard scarce game resources, so their ranges tend not to overlap.

Inter-cat relationships are not as formalised and immutable as they are in dog packs. Because they are subtle we might have trouble understanding them. Nevertheless they are genuine relationships, and when they break down the remedies can help.

♡ Try Beech for cats that cannot tolerate the presence of others, and spit and complain to show their displeasure.

♡ Choose Vine for very dominant cats that bully others.

♡ Select Centaury for submissive cats that tend not to fight back or resist.

♡ Chicory is for cats that like to keep their particular friends close by them, but reject the attentions of newcomers.

♡ Give Heather to cats that are desperate for any company and follow other cats around.

♡ Try Agrimony for sociable, easy-going animals that begin to look uneasy when they are on their own.

♡ Try Holly for cats that seem to show spite towards others, or get jealous if another cat steals affection from one of their feline or human companions.

♡ Choose Water Violet for cats that like their own company and sometimes find it hard to adjust when there are other cats around.

♡ Select Impatiens for cats that are in too much of a hurry to make friends.

♡ Use Mimulus for shy, timid cats that avoid the company of louder or more extrovert animals.

♡ Give Larch to cats that seem to lack the basic confidence needed to make a mark in cat society.

♡ Walnut is to help adjust to any changes in the cat's relationships.

♡ Choose Honeysuckle for a cat that has failed to adjust to a change in relationships and continually seeks out old associates, even if it means travelling a long way away from a new home.

Cats and people

Think for a minute about the different sorts of homes we provide for cats. On the one hand there is the farm cat, living a semi-wild existence off the rats and mice it catches. Then there is the alley cat – feral, but living a scavenger's life off the food that we donate or throw away. The apartment cat (a mainly US phenomenon) hardly ever goes out of the house. And the family cat puts up with the attentions of quick and clumsy toddlers, and stays a kitten into old age for the amusement of the children and their parents. Our habits and preferences have a huge impact on their way of life, yet cats cope very well with the different demands we place on them. Their flexibility is astonishing, especially when you compare them with other species.

Most social animals set up a fairly rigid dominance hierarchy. With dogs top dog is top dog. Leadership of the group is established by aggression and subsequent challenges are rare – which is why it is so easy to train a dog to accept us as permanent leader. Dominance between cats is far more fluid, and between similar animals can change from moment to moment without any obvious difference of opinion taking place. Cats always have the option to leave the relationship, because they are lone hunters and do not need the pack to survive. This flexibility allows us to leave them at home alone while we have a weekend break, but it also means that if we try to boss them around too much or fail to provide for them or frighten or mistreat them they will have no qualms about walking off. They can always get better accommodation somewhere else. There are then limits to what a cat will put up with. When we reach those limits the remedies can help cats cope with our sometimes unreasonable expectations. And we can and should take them ourselves as well, to help us view the relationship in a more even-handed way.

♡ Mimulus for the cat that has been frightened by a human, or Rock Rose where the reaction is real terror.

♡ The same fear remedies are also good for cats that were not handled as kittens and so never learned to trust people. You might need to add Holly for the fundamental suspicion that sometimes accompanies fear in such animals.

♡ Cherry Plum for a cat that has lost control of itself. An example of a Cherry Plum state in a cat might be where a play session with a trusted human has got out of hand. The cat suddenly feels vulnerable and in a moment lashes out at its human, then immediately after is frightened and confused by what it has done.

♡ Cerato for cats that depend on humans to help them make decisions. They lack confidence in themselves, and will look to their humans for confirmation before acting, as if checking that what they are going to do is acceptable.

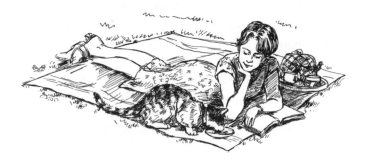

♡ Heather for cats that shamelessly seek out any and all human company, or Chicory for equally demanding cats that restrict their attentions to their close family and friends.

♡ Agrimony for class clown cats that enjoy playing the fool but seem ill at ease when left to their own devices.

♡ Willow for resentful cats that never seem content no matter how much is done for them.

♡ Vervain for enthusiastic cats that get over-excited when you play with them or when visitors arrive and so on.

Pregnancy

Inexperienced cat owners may only realise a queen is pregnant when they notice an increase in weight and a swelling tummy. But the first signs appear much earlier, about three weeks into the nine-week pregnancy, when the cat's nipples turn reddish pink and become more prominent. This is especially noticeable in first-time mothers. The queen's behaviour may also change as she begins to look at the world through the eyes of an expectant mother, and becomes softer and more affectionate. Nest-building happens in cats just as it does in birds and humans.

Pregnant cats eat more than usual. As well as providing extra food and some nesting materials, such as a cardboard box lined with newspaper, you can also be on hand with the remedies for when the going gets tough.

- ♡ Walnut will help the queen adjust to the various changes she is going through.

- ♡ For tiredness caused by the physical strain of the pregnancy, give Olive.

- ♡ Try Hornbeam where the cat seems energetic enough when actually called on to do something, but is lethargic and slow at first.

- ♡ Queens that become especially lazy and show no interest in even the mildest exercise might be encouraged with a few run-and-chase-me toys and the use of Wild Rose.

- ♡ Very occasionally queens suffer from nausea and a form of morning sickness. Add Crab Apple to the drinking water to help combat this.

Giving birth and after

At the end of the pregnancy the proud queen will usually produce three or four kittens. Single births are commoner in older queens, and at the other end of the scale a Persian in South Africa once gave birth to fourteen kittens, five of them stillborn. Cats give birth more easily than humans because each kitten in a litter is smaller and slighter in relation to its mother than human babies are to theirs. Queens usually manage very well by themselves and do not need the help of anxious humans. Nevertheless you should call the vet for advice if labour is prolonged and fruitless or the cat seems in pain.

Most cats need to rest for a day after giving birth, and should be allowed time and space to do this. New mothers will be more themselves by the second day, when they will have resumed their usual eating and drinking patterns.

Remedies that might help during labour and immediately afterwards include:

♡ Rescue Remedy to help keep mother calm.

♡ Olive where the mother cat seems worn out by the effort of having the kittens.

♡ Oak to encourage a cat that has struggled for a long time and has reached the limits of her endurance.

♡ Hornbeam or Wild Rose, as appropriate, to encourage effort in a cat that does not seem to be trying very hard.

♡ Star of Bethlehem for shock.

♡ Rock Rose for terror (this can apply to highly strung cats that panic when they see the first kitten arrive).

♡ Cherry Plum for the new mother that loses self-control and threatens to injure the kittens or herself.

♡ Walnut to help the queen adjust to the physical and emotional changes she is going through.

Neutering

There was once a popular theory that all queens should have at least one litter before being neutered. Thankfully this belief is dying out. Cat welfare groups agree that there are too many unwanted cats around already, and although strays can survive in the wild they do so at the expense of any local wildlife. Unless you have a very good reason not to you should consider having your cat neutered.

With modern techniques neutering is not dangerous or painful. Sometimes vets recommend it as a way of stopping inconvenient behaviour. Fertile females come into season several times a year and when they are in heat they call to every tom for miles around. The noise – and the sexual activity that ensues – can be quite spectacular, and is not to everyone's taste. Unneutered toms mark their territory by spraying pungent jets of urine on handy vertical surfaces such as walls, car wheels and chairs. They also get into more than their fair share of fights, both in competition for calling queens, and in order to back up their assertive odours.

Neutering solves these problems because a neutered queen no longer calls and a neutered tom, even if he still occasionally sprays, does not produce the same strong offensive odour. Neutered toms also move down the local pecking order, which means they do not have to fight to defend their position as much as their entire brothers.

The remedies can help anxious owners and cats cope with neutering.

♡ Take Pine if you feel guilty about having your cat neutered.

♡ Take Red Chestnut if you are overly worried about the operation hurting or doing some damage.

♡ Cats that get anxious whenever they are taken to the vet (perhaps due to early experiences with vaccinations and so on) can be helped with Mimulus or Rock Rose, or kept calm with doses of Rescue Remedy.

Moving house

Cats are territorial and social creatures. Their boundaries do not respect our walls and fences, but result from careful and continued negotiation between your cat and all the other cats in the neighbourhood. All the local cats know each other and know where they can go and when in order to avoid conflict. It should come as no surprise then that taking a cat away from its social milieu and its own territory and placing it in a totally new area does occasionally cause problems. Indeed, a house move is one of the most stressful events in a cat's life. To get an idea of how stressful, imagine how you would feel if you were suddenly taken away from your house and regular habits and inserted into a new neighbourhood, with no time to prepare, and without being consulted.

Fortunately the remedies can help ease your cat into its new environment.

♡ Give Walnut at once and then four times a day until the cat has settled in.

♡ Where the move has come as an especial shock, give Star of Bethlehem.

♡ For cats that seem to lose their confidence, and do not try to explore the new territory, select Larch.

♡ For cats that respond with fear, becoming anxious outside or away from you, select Mimulus. Aspen may also apply.

♡ Cats that abandon the new home and turn up on the doorstep of the old one can live more in the present if you give them Honeysuckle.

♡ Give Beech to cats that appear to dislike everything about the new neighbourhood.

♡ Cats that seem downcast and disheartened following a move can be given Gentian or Gorse, depending on the degree of despondency. If they go silent or complain all the time consider Willow or Heather as well.

New arrivals

Some cats can accept all kinds of changes in their home environment. Others are less accommodating, and one of the commonest problems animal behaviourists see is the cat that will not tolerate a new arrival in the household. Usually the newcomer is another cat, but it can also be a new baby, a house guest or your boyfriend or girlfriend.

When introducing a new cat into your house it is a good idea to go slowly and take precautions. Start by keeping the new cat

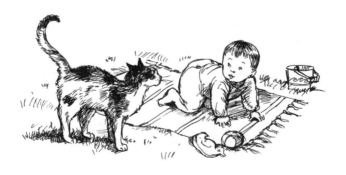

in a room by itself, so that the old cat knows it is there and can smell it, but can't attack. An indoor pen can also be useful, allowing you to let the two cats see and smell each other without the risk of a fight breaking out. You can leave the new cat in different parts of the house, safe in its pen, so as to underline its right to be anywhere in the old cat's territory. You can even feed the cats side by side, separated by the cage, so that they get used to sharing personal space.

When you do allow the cats to get within clawing distance of each other you need to be around just in case things get out of hand. Do not interfere too early, however, as the threats and sideswipes are part of the process of establishing a relationship. Try not to give your old cat an excuse to be jealous. Do not be seen to be too friendly to the new arrival until the older cat has accepted it. If you have allowed them to acclimatise to each other the first face-to-face confrontation should not present too many problems.

Much the same approach can be taken with the cat that responds badly to a new human in the house. Keep the cat in a pen while the newcomer is in the room. Adults can put out the cat's food for a time as a bribe, and you can encourage toddlers and children to keep calm around the cat. Never allow children to reinforce fear-based aggression by mistreating or frightening the cat in any way.

The remedies can also be useful where things do not go as smoothly as you might have wished.

♡ Walnut is the remedy to help cats adjust to changes in the environment.

♡ Where fear is the main reason for aggression towards newcomers, use Mimulus to give the cat more courage. The same remedy could also help cats that run away from strangers.

♡ Jealous cats that dislike having their existing web of relationships disrupted could be helped with Holly or Chicory.

♡ Relatively dominant cats that cannot tolerate newcomers and are continually attacking and hitting out at them could be helped with Beech or Vine.

♡ Try Cherry Plum for cats that attack in a frenzy, with no self-control, and then as suddenly stop and appear confused, perhaps engaging in displacement activities such as grooming.

♡ Cats that withdraw from contact with the family following the arrival of a newcomer might be helped with Water Violet, Chicory or Willow. Mimulus is also a possibility where there is fear.

♡ Cats that whinge and moan a lot to get attention could be helped with Heather.

Rescue cats

You might think that the cat you get from a cat sanctuary or rescue home has had to be rescued from something. Certainly some animals have been mistreated in the past and may need a lot of love and attention before they will begin to respond to their new owners. But this is not always true. Sometimes cats are 'rescued' from perfectly normal and enjoyable lives as strays. Their problem lies in the present – dealing with new relationships and a change of home and diet, not to mention the unaccustomed company of humans.

The single most used remedy for rescue cats is Rescue Remedy. But with a little thought you can make a more focused choice and so be more helpful to the cat.

♡ If a cat has been mistreated or has suffered past traumas, give Star of Bethlehem.

♡ If a cat is finding it hard to adjust to a change in circumstances or owner, give Walnut.

♡ If a cat has been institutionalised at the rescue home and now lacks the confidence to explore its new surroundings, give Larch.

♡ If a cat is fearful of people or new situations, give Mimulus.

♡ Where fear is outright terror give Rock Rose, and where it seems general and there is no specific trigger try Aspen instead.

♡ Give Honeysuckle if the cat seems uninterested in its new life and repeats behaviour more appropriate to life at or prior to the rescue home.

Cat shows

Historians trace the birth of the cat show back to a fair held in England in 1598. Serious cat fanciers show pure-bred cats, but most shows have a 'household pet' class where healthier and more robust moggies compete on personality and looks. Shows tend to be more fun for owners than they are for cats. Nevertheless, you can do a few things before the event to help your cat get through the day more comfortably.

First, make sure your cat is used to its carry box, and used to travelling in the car. Ideally it should associate being in the box and travelling with nice things like food, attention and play. It will not relax on the way to the show if it links car journeys with vets and vaccinations. Second, get the cat used to being handled by strangers. You might have to enlist the help of friends and neighbours to do this, but at least you will avoid the embarrassment of watching your nervous puss attacking the cat show judges. Third, use the remedies to help get your cat – and you – through the day with the minimum of angst.

♡ Cats that get nervous or upset at the show can be given Rescue Remedy.

♡ Give Vervain to lively animals that get over-excited and want to join in right away.

♡ Cats that seem fearful or cowed can be helped with Mimulus.

♡ Consider Cherry Plum in addition to Mimulus for cats that lose their composure and lash out.

Old age

Cats have been known to live into their thirties, but a more likely life expectancy is sixteen or seventeen. As they get older they suffer from many of the same afflictions as humans. Hair loss is more likely, as are dental problems, and hearing and sight both start to fade. Cats that were once outdoor, adventurous types start to spend more time sitting around indoors. They may be reluctant to go outside in the cold to urinate and defecate, or suffer from incontinence. Either cause can lead to uncharacteristic accidents around the house.

Sometimes their attitudes harden along with their arteries, and they show less tolerance towards kittens and anything else 'new-fangled' that might disrupt their orderly lives. This includes new foods – most cats will be fussy given the chance, but the older the cat the more likely this is. Other cats, however, seem to welcome youngsters and new toys and foods and in fact remain kittenish and curious right into old age. Here too they are just like people.

♡ Cats that are very set in their ways and get irritable when unexpected things happen can be helped with Beech.

♡ Walnut helps adjust to difficult changes at any age, and is also good for easing your cat through the different stages of life.

♡ Try giving Olive or Hornbeam to cats that seem tired all the time.

♡ Try Wild Rose for cats that lose their enthusiasm for life, or stop grooming themselves through lack of interest.

♡ Cats that cope well most of the time but seem to lose heart and confidence when things get too much for them could be helped with Elm.

♡ Oak is the remedy for those brave old plodders who keep going at the same even pace until they break down.

♡ Old cats that sleep all the time, so much so that they barely seem anchored to life at all, might benefit from Clematis.

♡ 'Forgetting' to use the litter tray and a general lack of attention to what is going on around them can also be helped with Clematis.

♡ Cats losing their hair and physical condition can get depressed. Try Crab Apple to help them accept themselves as they are.

Common ailments

Some cat illnesses are very serious and can prove fatal. You need to be aware of the symptoms so that you can take prompt action. Always consult a vet if you think that your cat might be suffering from any of the following illnesses:

♡ Cat 'flu
Cat 'flu is the short name for feline upper respiratory tract disease. There are two variants. The more serious and potentially fatal variety is feline viral rhinotrachcitis. The symptoms include sneezing and coughing and a runny nose. The less serious variety of 'flu is feline calcivirus.

♡ Feline immunodeficiency virus
The feline immunodeficiency virus FIV is the cat equivalent to HIV in humans. It attacks the cat's immune system, and so compromises its ability to fight infection. As a result opportunistic infections – other viruses and bacteria – can attack the cat. You can't catch HIV from FIV-infected cats.

♡ Feline infectious anaemia
Feline infectious anaemia is characterised by fatigue and anaemia. The cause is a blood-born parasite that destroys red blood cells.

♡ Feline infectious enteritis
This is a serious infection that causes severe diarrhoea and vomiting, accompanied by fever. You need to get immediate medical help if you suspect a case of feline infectious enteritis, because there is a serious risk of dehydration and death.

♡ Feline infectious peritonitis
Feline infectious peritonitis is characterised by jaundice, diarrhoea and vomiting, rapid weight loss and fatigue. Fluid may collect in the abdomen as well, although this does not happen in all cases.

♡ Feline leukaemia
Feline leukaemia is caused by a virus. The main sign of

infection is anaemia, and because the virus attacks the immune system a range of other symptoms may appear.

♡ Toxoplasmosis
Humans can catch this disease from the faeces of small animals like rabbits, guinea pigs and cats. Adults who catch it may get a slight fever or experience no symptoms at all, but it can cause very serious conditions in human foetuses. This is why doctors and midwives advise pregnant women to avoid contact with cats and cat faeces. In cats toxoplasmosis causes a variety of symptoms including runny noses, weight loss, diarrhoea and respiratory infections.

On one level illness is caused by bacteria and viruses, and when a cat becomes ill you should get medical help to treat the physical agents of the disease. However, vets will tell you that some cats fall ill at the drop of hat while others remain hale and hearty through every epidemic. Bach Flower Remedies do not treat the actual disease, but you should take time to think about the remedies, and focus on this question: why did *my* cat get sick when it came across this germ?

♡ Where there has been a change in the cat's life give Walnut to help it adjust. The change might not be obvious to you. Maybe you have a new job and get home an hour later than normal. You are no longer there at playtime, and that could be a big change to the cat.

♡ Walnut is also useful if there is some upset in the house – perhaps arguments between you and your partner – and this influence is putting your cat under stress.

♡ Consider the way the animal is responding to the illness. A cat that follows you around whining for attention is probably in a Chicory or Heather state. This state could actually be the underlying cause of the illness and not a symptom at all. A cat that mopes in the corner feeling sorry for itself will need Willow, while one that refuses to rest and goes about its round in a dogged, determined manner may well be ill *because* it has refused to rest. In this case give Oak.

Under the following headings we list some of the commoner physical symptoms that cats experience. Suggestions for possible Bach Flower Remedies are given, but they are only suggestions. Any of the remedies could apply to your cat when it has a physical problem. You need to look at the cat not the disease, and of course use a specific treatment for the disease itself at the same time. Don't forget to take the remedies yourself so that you can be a better nurse. Look again at page 43 for some suggestions. Finally, keep the Rescue Remedy handy for both of you for those emergencies where there is no time to think about how you and your cat feel.

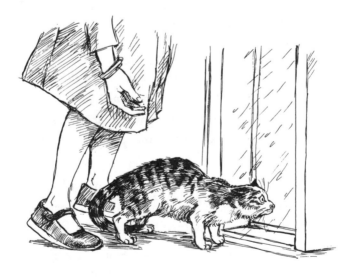

Skin problems

Cats share a number of common skin problems with humans, including eczema, abscesses, warts and alopecia (hair loss). In addition there are some problems that are peculiar to cats, such as stud tail, in which a greasy oil appears on the tail, causing fur to mat and come away.

In addition to seeking the advice of the vet, who will be able to diagnose the exact condition that your cat is suffering from, the following remedies are particularly worth bearing in mind.

♡ Rescue Cream – this is good for many types of skin disorder. In cases of eczema, however, try a little on one area of the skin first, since some eczemas respond badly to the application of any type of cream.

♡ Crab Apple – this is the cleansing remedy, and will help any cat that feels contaminated or unclean or seems upset at the change in its appearance. It can be combined with Rescue Remedy and used diluted in water in any cleansing routine.

♡ Impatiens – this will help cats that seem to be irritated and agitated by itchy patches.

♡ Cherry Plum – where itchiness or pain leads to the cat losing its self-possession and lashing out at you or biting or scratching or grooming itself to the point of self-injury.

♡ Walnut – this may be useful where you suspect that something in the environment or a change in the cat's lifestyle is causing the problem.

Parasites

Parasites are animals that live off other animals. They can be divided into external parasites, such as fleas and lice, and internal, such as the various kind of worms. Like all higher animals, cats can harbour both types. Cat fleas are the most common, but any kind of parasite can infest a cat given the right conditions.

Treatment with Bach Flower Remedies alone is unlikely to get rid of parasites. Use a conventional approach, then, such as proprietary mixes or preparations from the vet. If you prefer to avoid using insecticides and conventional de-wormers you might consider using aromatherapy or herbal medicines. But ask an expert first – incorrect use of either can kill your cat. You can still use Bach Flower Remedies to help the cat feel better within itself, so that it is less bothered by the infestation and by the treatment you use to deal with it.

♡ Give Crab Apple if your cat seems to feel unhappy about the parasites, especially where it is continually scratching or grooming to get rid of fleas or ticks.

♡ Add Cherry Plum where excessive grooming or scratching threatens to injure the cat.

♡ Ticks are external parasites that lock into the cat's skin, usually around its ears. They can be stunned with Rescue Remedy before being removed with tweezers. Do this very carefully so as to avoid leaving part of the tick inside the cat. (This is the one occasion where the brandy in the stock bottle is an active ingredient. The alcohol paralyses the tick and makes it easier to remove it cleanly. The Rescue itself helps deal with any distress the cat feels during the procedure.)

There is evidence that parasites are more common in unhappy, unhealthy cats. This is certainly the case with lice, which only rarely afflict healthy cats. Use of the remedies in everyday life can help your cat stay balanced and healthy, and in this way help to reduce the chance of future infestations.

Eye problems

Cats' eyes share common features with the eyes of all mammals, so it is no surprise that many of the problems common in humans are also present in cats, including conjunctivitis, glaucoma, cataracts and failing eyesight in old age. Signs that all is not well with the eyes include epiphora (a discharge from the tear ducts running down either side of the muzzle), red-rimmed eyes, or the appearance of a film covering the inner corners. The film is the cat's third eyelid, called a *haw*, usually you can't see it when the cat is healthy.

Untreated infections or wounds can cause permanent damage to the eyesight, so get a vet to look at any persistent soreness or other symptoms in this area. The vet can't do anything about the failing of sight in old age, of course, but cats compensate well for failing sight by making more use of their wonderful sense of smell.

♡ Give Gentian to a cat that seems despondent due to an eye problem, or try Willow if it looks particularly sorry for itself.

♡ If you are using eye baths or otherwise washing out the eyes, try adding a few drops of Crab Apple and/or Rescue Remedy to the clean water. (Never use neat remedies near the eyes.) Salt solutions are often recommended for bathing eyes: add half a teaspoon of salt and a couple of drops of remedies to every pint of distilled water.

♡ Very visual cats that begin to avoid challenging
situations due to an eye problem can be helped with
Larch.

Nose problems

Dogs are famous for having sensitive noses, but in fact the cat's
nose is more sensitive still. The nose is a delicate organ, and
cats can get very miserable if it is not in good working order.

Treat a snuffly cat in the same way you would a small baby
with a cold. First, see page 86 and get proper medical attention
if you suspect a genuine case of 'flu – this is serious enough to
warrant calling out an expert. Do your best to keep the nose
clear by gently bathing it with warm water and wiping away the
softened mucus. You can also smooth a little petroleum jelly
into the sore nose – again, this will sound familiar to the parents of non-feline babies.

Causes of a runny nose include allergies and various kinds of
bacterial and viral infections. Some cats go off their food when
they have a blocked nose. This is not usually something to
worry about, and their appetite will return once the underlying
problem has been dealt with.

♡ When cleaning mucus from the nose, add Rescue
Remedy and/or Crab Apple to the warm water.

♡ A small amount of Rescue Cream can be used instead of
petroleum jelly to stop the nose from drying out and
help keep it clear.

♡ You might give Hornbeam, Wild Rose, Gentian, Gorse,
Clematis and other remedies to cats that are off their
food, depending on how you read their current state of
mind.

Ear problems

Cats have excellent hearing and hear at a much higher register than dogs. Hearing declines with age, however, and white cats (particularly those with blue eyes) are inclined to suffer from congenital deafness. When a cat has one blue eye and one of another colour the deafness often occurs on one side only.

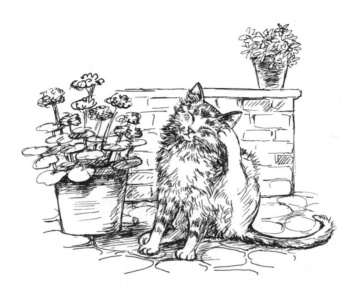

When a cat starts shaking its head and scratching at its ear there is a good chance that it has a problem with its ear. Possible causes include parasites, the presence of a foreign body, and an infection of some kind, whether from a bacterial illness or a fungus. If the middle or inner ear are affected there may be loss of balance as well.

♡ Give Crab Apple if the cat seems particularly bothered by an ear infection. If the vet advises warmed olive oil to help clear wax from the ears try adding a couple of drops of Crab Apple to the oil before using it.

♡ Swelling around the ears may be helped with Rescue Cream. This contains Rescue Remedy and Crab Apple, and can be applied to the affected area, as many times as seems necessary.

♡ Scleranthus is the remedy most associated with dizziness and loss of balance, because it is indicated when a fluctuating state occurs. Give it where the cat seems uncertain and indecisive, and consult the vet.

♡ If the head-shaking and scratching is out of control give Cherry Plum. This especially applies if the cat is in danger of causing itself injury.

Coughs

Cats are as likely to get coughs as we are, and for as many reasons. Viral infection is one possibility, especially from the cat 'flu virus (see page 86), but other causes include anything from the minor (inhaling cigarette smoke) to the potentially serious (tumours). Parasite infestation, bronchitis, asthma and allergies can all cause coughing. Seek the advice of a vet where coughing is persistent or serious or where there are other symptoms such as a high temperature or nasal discharge.

When selecting Bach Flower Remedies for a coughing cat, consider how it seems to feel about the cough, and the way it reacts.

♡ Give Rescue Remedy to ease immediate distress.

♡ Use Crab Apple as a cleanser, especially where the cat is coughing up phlegm and seems distressed by this.

♡ Choose Agrimony for cats that are obviously ill but remain playful, or Oak for those that carry on with their usual business and refuse to give in.

♡ Choose from Wild Rose, Gentian and Gorse for animals that seem to give up when they are ill.

♡ Give Olive if the coughing is persistent so that the cat cannot sleep its usual sixteen hours and seems tired.

♡ Select Chicory or Heather for cats that become very clingy.

♡ Try Willow for cats that retire to a favourite corner and mope.

Other respiratory problems

Cats suffer from as many respiratory problems as humans do, including asthma, pneumonia and the cat's version of the 'flu (see page 86). All have been linked to stress, so the remedies are an obvious helper to use alongside whatever other treatment the vet recommends.

♡ Panic makes an acute asthma attack worse. Rescue Remedy has proved useful as it helps keep the cat calm and so aids breathing.

♡ Impatiens may help restless, agitated cats suffering from pneumonia.

♡ Crab Apple is the cleansing remedy, and can help cats that seem to be contaminated with phlegm and fever.

Mouth and dental problems

Cats that have a problem with their mouths may exhibit one or more of the following symptoms: excessive salivation, apparent discomfort or over-care while eating, scratching or pawing at the mouth, and bad breath. Inflammation of the gums or the lining of the mouth can be caused by infection or by dental problems. The latter are less common in cats than in people because cats are not especially fond of sugar, but they do happen, so consider consulting a vet for a dental examination.

The best way to avoid problems is good dental hygiene. Use an extra-soft child's toothbrush dipped in salty water and gently brush your cat's teeth once a week. Ask the vet to check the teeth and gums every year. Vets can descale teeth to remove any build up of tartar if this should prove necessary.

- ♡ Where recurrent ulcers occur or the cat seems especially prone to tartar build-up, try Crab Apple for its cleansing properties.

- ♡ Impatiens can help calm a cat agitated by toothache. Rescue Remedy is good for this as well.

Obesity

Cats are self-regulating, which means that left to their own devices they will not over-eat and will not become overweight. In human society, however, we do not leave them to their own devices. We see the offer of food as a sign of love and care, and the temptation to give treats to our cats can be overwhelming. Food manufacturers try to maximise sales and customer loyalty by making pet foods more palatable. Some cats can't resist and eat everything in the bowl every time it is filled. The combination of indulgent owners and artificially tasty food is a serious problem for cats. Unable to play or even move around with any comfort, the fat cat is a prisoner of its own body, and obesity is a factor in various illnesses and physical malfunctions from skin problems and arthritis to diabetes and liver and heart failure.

When trying to help an overweight cat start by consulting the vet to rule out the possibility of a physical cause such as a thyroid problem. The vet will be able to advise you on the optimum diet for your cat's breed, size, age and metabolic rate. This done, take a good hard look at yourself and at the things you are feeding your cat. Include treats and extras and write it all down. Cut out everything that goes beyond the vet's recommendations, and make up your mind to stick to the limit you set. You need to be honest with yourself if you are going to help your cat, and you can use the remedies as well, especially on yourself if you are the guilty party. Think about the following, then, for you and your cat:

♡ Chestnut Bud for failing to learn from past experiences.

♡ Chicory for the kind of possessive love that buys love and attention by fussing and caring too much.

♡ Walnut to help resist outside influences (for the cat, your offer of treats; for you, the appeal of the latest cat treat advert).

♡ Red Chestnut if you are afraid that your cat will starve if you cut down its food intake to the level recommended by your vet.

♡ Centaury if you keep giving in to your cat, or Agrimony if you will do anything to keep the peace, and continue to feed your cat rather than put up with its apparently urgent requests for more food.

♡ Larch if you expect to fail and feel that you are not strong-willed enough to help your cat cut down.

If you feel your cat is missing its little treats give more time and attention and play sessions instead. Time is more valuable than food when it comes to showing love, and shared fun and exercise will help increase the bond between you.

Vomiting

Most cats vomit occasionally. Causes vary from fur balls and undigested or contaminated food right up to infections and potentially serious diseases of the liver, pancreas and kidney. Usually cats vomit up whatever is troubling them right away, and after you have cleaned up the results your cat will get on with its day without any ill-effects. If your cat vomits more than once, however, consider imposing a 24-hour fast. Make sure you provide plenty of fresh drinking water and see a vet if the problem continues.

You should go to the vet at once if vomiting is severe or frequent or comes accompanied with other symptoms. In severe cases there is a risk of dehydration since water taken in will not stay down long enough to be ingested. In these circumstances your cat needs skilled help as soon as possible. While waiting you can help by spooning in a mixture of water, sugar and a little salt.

In all cases of vomiting the remedies can be used to help, although in severe cases they should never be given neat as they are preserved in brandy and can make things worse.

♡ Give diluted Rescue Remedy to calm distressed cats.

♡ Select Crab Apple for cats that seem to be trying to clear something out of their systems, and for those that seem particularly keen to avoid soiling themselves.

♡ Cherry Plum helps where vomiting is uncontrolled and explosive, or where the cat loses its self-control.

♡ Water Violet or Mimulus may apply where the patient hides itself away and vomits in secret.

♡ Give Olive if the cat seems weak and shaky.

Other digestion problems

Cats can suffer from a wide range of digestive problems. Symptoms such as a lack of appetite may indicate fur balls – knots of fur swallowed during the cat's regular grooming of itself – or more serious problems such as a disease of the pancreas. Eating more roughage solves most cases of constipation and a 24-hour fast deals with the majority of diarrhoea cases, but again both may be symptomatic of chronic illness.

The vast majority of digestive problems are stress-related in one way or another, and the Bach Flower Remedies can be particularly effective in this area. As usual they should be selected for the emotional state of the cat and not for any physical symptoms.

♡ Fear is a potent cause of stress in cats, and can lead to digestive upsets. Think about Mimulus, Aspen or Red Chestnut depending on the type of fear concerned.

♡ Cats that put themselves under stress might benefit from Impatiens, Vervain or Oak. Select the remedy that is closest to your cat's current state of mind: Impatiens for impatient types that want everything to happen five minutes ago, Vervain for enthusiasts that can't switch off, and Oak for cats that refuse to rest, struggling on at the same steady pace regardless of circumstances.

♡ Crab Apple can be good for cats that are clearly bothered by diarrhoea or constipation.

♡ Lack of appetite may be helped with Wild Rose, Clematis or Hornbeam – again, the right remedy depends on the individual cat.

Genito-urinary problems

A vaginal discharge often signals genital problems in female cats. Take queens with this symptom to the vet for examination, and do so as a matter of urgency if the queen is pregnant. In entire males one potentially serious problem is orchitis, or inflamed testicles. Causes vary from infection to injury, and again any tom suffering from painful testicles should be taken to the vet for an examination.

Urinary problems include cystitis and kidney disease. Look for symptoms such as blood in the urine, and cats straining to pass water or passing water very frequently. Once again it is important to get veterinary advice in these situations, and the remedies also have a part to play.

♡ Wipe away vaginal discharges with a weak solution of Crab Apple and antiseptic in warm water.

♡ Cats in pain due to swollen testicles or cystitis can become agitated and lash out. Impatiens will help keep them calm, and Cherry Plum may also be used. Rescue Remedy, which contains both these remedies, is another alternative.

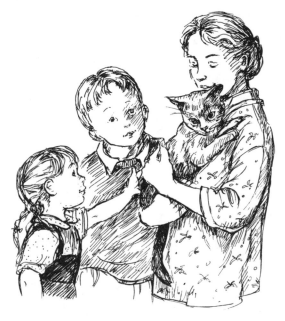

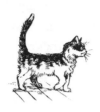

Part Three

Other natural therapies

Many other therapies can help cats. Some are well known and widely available, such as orthodox veterinary care and herbal medicine. But some of the less famous techniques are well worth exploring, especially as a combination of approaches often turns out to be more effective than any one in isolation.

Bach Flower Remedies are widely used by complementary therapists of various disciplines, occasionally as a more appropriate alternative to their main therapy, but usually as a helpful complementary aid, the two therapies used in tandem so as to approach a single problem from two directions at once. Bach Flower Remedies do not react or interfere with other treatments, which makes them especially well adapted to complementing other therapies in this way. (Note however that the alcohol in the remedies may react with some medicines. Always dilute the remedies where possible, and consult your vet if in doubt.) And because the remedy drops can be given in between actual sessions with a therapist, they are a good way of maintaining a sense of continual progress.

We have not attempted to list all the possible approaches to emotional health that exist, or to give a full account of each therapy. Instead what follows is an overview of some useful approaches, most of them similar to Bach Flower Remedies in that they approach health holistically. This means they take account of spiritual and emotional issues as well as physical symptoms. In general, these therapies work by stimulating a healthier and more vibrant flow of energy, hoping in this way to restore harmony to the whole and reactivate the body's own healing resources. We have listed some good general guides to each therapy and/or a contact address so that you can find out more about it.

Acupuncture

An ancient Chinese medical technique, based on the Tao philosophy of yin/yang energy flow. In Tao philosophy vital energy (chi or qi) flows along meridians or energy pathways in the body. This flow is either masculine, active and positive(yin), or feminine, passive and negative(yang). Ill health occurs if yin and yang are out of balance or the chi is blocked in some way. Treatment involves tapping into the flow of energy and dispelling the blockage. The energy within the meridian is stimulated and this in turn encourages a return of yin/yang balance and restored health. Traditionally practitioners work by inserting fine needles into the skin at specific points, although some use heat or fingertip pressure.

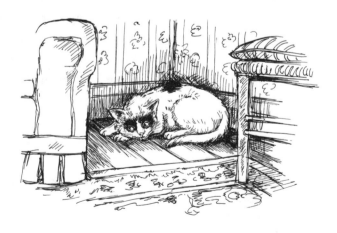

Acupuncture should only ever be carried out by a qualified acupuncturist. If you feel it could help your cat ask your vet to refer you to a competent person.

♡ For more information see *Principles of Acupuncture* by Angela Hicks (Thorsons, London); or contact The British Acupuncture Council, 63 Jeddo Road, London, W12 9HQ, UK.

Aromatherapy

Aromatherapy uses the aromatic essential oils of plants. Different oils are indicated for different ailments and are used to restore both physical and emotional harmony. They are also used as an aid to relaxation.

Practitioners usually administer the oils by diluting them into a carrier oil and then massaging them into the skin. They can also be heated using a burner, which fills the room with a pleasant and therapeutic aroma, or added to bath water, creams or lotions. In some circumstances they can be given orally, but this should only be done under the advice of a qualified aromatherapist. Many of the oils used in aromatherapy can be poisonous if taken internally.

Again, you are advised to contact a vet in the first instance to get a referral to a qualified person who has experience in treating animals. You should never give essential oils by mouth without consulting an expert, and aromatherapy should not be used if your cat is already on drugs – doing so can lead to liver failure. Finally, remember that cats will lick oils off their skin if they can reach them.

♡ For more information see *Veterinary Aromatherapy* by Nelly Grosjean (The CW Daniel Co, Saffron Walden);

or contact The Aromatherapy Organisations Council,
PO Box 19834, London, SE25 6WF, UK.

Chinese herbalism

Like acupuncture, Chinese herbalism is an ancient medical system that goes back thousands of years. It aims to treat both mind and body, and practitioners choose herbs constitutionally rather than for specific ailments.

The practitioner of Chinese herbalism uses a great variety of different herbs. Some, such as ginseng, are readily available and do not cause unwanted effects, but others are harder to get hold of and may make things worse if you use them incorrectly. For this reason you should consult a practitioner in the first instance rather than try to pick the right herbs for your cat yourself, and you should not give herbs to a cat that is already on drugs.

> ♡ For more information see *Principles of Chinese Herbal
> Medicine* by John Hicks (Thorsons, London) or
> *Chinese Medicine – The Web that has no Weaver* by
> Ted Kaptchuk (Rider, London); or contact the Register
> of Chinese Herbal Medicine, PO Box 400, Wembley
> HA9 9NZ, UK.

Chiropractic

Chiropractic (sometimes referred to incorrectly as chiropractice) treats problems with the muscles and joints. Practitioners seek to adjust abnormalities in the musculo-skeletal system. This relieves pressure on nerves that could if left untreated lead to many other forms of disease.

In addition to traditional chiropractic there is a newer version available called McTimoney chiropractic. This uses a set of movements perfected by a well-known teacher and practitioner, John McTimoney. Practitioners of both forms of the therapy can treat animals, subject to referral from a vet.

♡ For more information on 'classical' chiropractic contact The British Chiropractic Association, 29 Whitley Street, Reading, RG2 0EG, UK; for information on McTimoney chiropractic contact The McTimoney Chiropractic Association, 21 High Street, Eynsham, Oxfordshire, OX8 1HE, UK.

Healing

Healing does not use pills or potions, but relies on simple contact between a healer's hands and the animal. It is based on the understanding that everything in life, whether physical matter or spiritual force, is a form of energy. Healing encourages the free flow of energy between the higher self – understood as the life force of the individual – and the individual's physical and emotional being. The healer uses herself as a channel, tapping into the spiritual energy of life and directing its flow to the individual being healed. Recipients may feel heat emanating from the hands of the healer, and a sense of peace and relaxation or relief from pain. Successive healing sessions aim to encourage a permanent return of this vital flow of energy, which in turn brings about an improved state of health.

♡ For more information contact The National Federation of Spiritual Healers, Old Manor Farm Studio, Church Street, Sunbury-on-Thames, Middlesex, TW16 6RG, UK.

Herbal medicine

The use of medicinal herbs is thousands of years old but reached its peak in the 16th century. Nicholas Culpepper, who lived then, remains one of the best known herbalists – his famous book on herbalism is still in print. Herbal medicines re-create balance in the body and treat the whole person, rather than an isolated disease. They can be used as preventative as well as curative medicines.

You can take medicinal herbs in several different ways. You will find tablets, powders and liquid preparations in the shops, and dried herbs can be made into infusions similar to tea. Some herbal medicines have been prepared especially for the home treatment of cats and other domestic animals, but seek advice before using them if your cat is already on medication.

> ♡ For more information see *A Guide to Herbal Remedies* by Mark Evans (The CW Daniel Co, Saffron Walden); or *Complete Guide to Modern Herbalism* by Simon Mills (Thorsons, London); or contact The National Institute of Medical Herbalists, 56 Longbrook Street, Exeter, Devon, EX4 6AH, UK.

Homoeopathy

Homoeopathy was founded by Samuel Hahnemann, an 18th century German doctor. He found that a small dose of a substance that was known to produce certain symptoms would help the body fight off a disease with the same symptoms. This is known as the principle of 'like curing like'. For example, the homoeopathic remedy Alium Cepa is indicated for colds which cause running eyes and nose. It is made from onions, which will of course produce the symptoms the homoeopathic preparation treats.

Homoeopathy uses the healing properties of plants, minerals and animal products, all in minute doses. It treats the whole person, and takes account of individual symptoms as well as personal characteristics. Thus a homoeopathic remedy reflects the constitution or personality of the recipient as well as the illness itself.

Homoeopathic medicines go through a process of potentisation which involves vigorous shaking between dilutions. This is called succussion. The more stages of succussion a remedy goes through the more potent it becomes. This means that homoeopathic medicines come in different strengths, the most usual being 6c and 30c. You can buy 6c remedies over the counter, and you will find preparations aimed specifically at cats and other animals. There are also plenty of homoeopathically-trained vets who offer an alternative to orthodox medical care, even for serious illnesses. To get in contact with one go first to your own vet and ask for a referral.

♡ For more information see *Homoeopathy in Veterinary Practice* by K J Biddis, *A Veterinary Materia Medica and Clinical Repertory* by George Macleod, and *Cats: Homoeopathic Remedies* by G Macleod (all The CW Daniel Co, Saffron Walden); or contact The British Homoeopathic Association, 27A Devonshire Street, London, W1N 1RJ, UK, or the Society of Homoeopaths, 2 Artizan Road, Northampton, NN1 4HU, UK.

Osteopathy

Osteopathy is related to chiropractic – in fact the person who first developed chiropractic was a practising osteopath – and like that therapy involves manipulating the body in order to improve the functioning of its systems, tissues and organs. It is a holistic approach that focuses on the structure of the body, and treatment aims to bring about a return of vital energy and life force within the entire being.

In the UK osteopaths are regulated by law under the General Osteopathic Council. Osteopathy is widely accepted by orthodox medical practitioners, and referrals to osteopaths are becoming more common. You will need to go to your vet first if you feel that your cat might benefit from this approach.

♡ For more information see *Introductory Guide to Osteopathy* by Edward Triance (Thorsons, London); or contact The Osteopathy Information Service, PO Box 2074, Reading, RG1 4YR, UK.

Reflexology

The principle behind reflexology – also known as reflex zone therapy – is similar to that of acupuncture, in that it is based on the concept of channels, or meridians, that allow energy to flow through the body. Reflexologists consider illness to be the result of congestion of these channels, the congestion being caused by negative mental states or stress and tension. To relieve the person's ill-health they seek to restore a free flow of energy along the channels.

The feet are believed to be particularly sensitive and responsive because the body's energy flows from head to foot. Reflexologists concentrate on massaging and applying pressure to areas of the feet that are linked to different parts of the body via the energy channels. This helps the individual to relax and stimulates the related areas and body organs, releasing the energy block and allowing the return of a positive state of health.

Reflexology is available for cats as well, but referral from a vet will be required before the therapist can start work.

♡ For more information see *Reflexology: a step by step guide* by Peijian Shen (Gaia Books, London); or contact The Association of Reflexologists, 27 Old Gloucester Street, London, WC1 3XX, UK.

Veterinary care

Natural therapies can provide excellent results, but most of them will not by themselves replace orthodox veterinary care. Registration with a vet is vital if you want to be sure that your cat is going to remain healthy and well. Your vet is a qualified medical physician who will be able to examine, diagnose and advise on the appropriate treatment for all kinds of condition. He or she will be able to perform blood tests, X-rays and scans to determine exactly what the problem is, and carry out surgery where that is necessary. Interventions like this may save your cat's life.

Vets are also well placed to refer you on to other practitioners who specialise in specific areas of treating animals. This may include referral to qualified complementary practitioners. Generally speaking bona fide complementary practitioners will need to know that you have consulted a vet before they can begin treatment, and they will also want the vet to know about what they are doing. The different approaches of orthodox and holistic medicine, often diametrically opposed in their philosophy, actually go together extremely well on a practical level. Make a friend of your vet, then – and if yours turns out to be entirely against complementary medicine, find another more sympathetic to your own outlook.

Further reading

On Bach Flower Remedies

(The books listed here are all published by The C W Daniel Co., Saffron Walden, unless stated otherwise. You can order them from your local book shop or direct from the Bach Centre – see page 114 for the address.)

- ♡ *Bach Flower Remedies for Animals* by Judy Howard and Stefan Ball – the most authoritative work on using the remedies to help animals, this can be used in conjunction with the present book. It contains information on the philosophical basis of using the remedies with animals and a guide to selection that can be applied to any type of animal. There are also dozens of genuine case histories to inspire you.

- ♡ *The Twelve Healers and Other Remedies* by Dr Edward Bach – Dr Bach's final word on his discovery explains in simple terms what the remedies are for.

- ♡ *Bach Flower Remedies Step by Step* by Judy Howard – a simple general introduction to the remedies provides all the information you need to start using them.

- ♡ *The Bach Remedies Workbook* by Stefan Ball – an interactive course that uses games, quizzes and other activities to teach the system.

- ♡ *Principles of Bach Flower Therapy* by Stefan Ball (Thorsons, 1999) – covers all the basic principles of the therapy, including how the healing process works.

- ♡ *Questions and Answers* by John Ramsell – the questions that are most commonly asked, answered by the world's leading authority on the remedies.

- ♡ *Handbook of the Bach Flower Remedies* by Phillip Chancellor – hundreds of case studies collected from early editions of the Bach Centre's newsletter.

- ♡ *Bach Flower Remedies for Women* by Judy Howard – covers all the major stages in a woman's life, with suggestions for using the remedies to help from cradle to grave.

♡ *Bach Flower Remedies for Men* by Stefan Ball – the companion volume to Women deals with everything from school exams to sex, work and retirement.

♡ *Growing Up with Bach Flower Remedies* by Judy Howard – how to select remedies for children of all ages.

♡ *Heal Thyself* by Dr Edward Bach – Dr Bach's philosophy of healing, told in his own words.

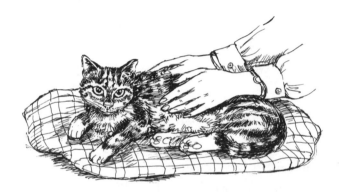

♡ *The Original Writings of Edward Bach* edited by John Ramsell and Judy Howard – a selection of Dr Bach's writings, some of them never before published.

♡ *The Medical Discoveries of Edward Bach, Physician* by Nora Weeks – the story of Dr Bach's working life, told by the woman who worked with him as he discovered and completed the system of flower remedies.

♡ *The Bach Flower Gardener* by Stefan Ball – how to use the remedies to help plants, illustrated with many real-life case studies.

On cats

♡ Allport, Richard, *Heal Your Cat the Natural Way*, Mitchell Beazley, London, 1997

♡ Fogle, Bruce, *The Cat's Mind*, Pelham Books, London, 1991

♡ Lorenz, Konrad, *On Aggression*, Methuen & Co, London, 1966

♡ Masson, Jeffrey and McCarthy, Susan, *When Elephants Weep*, Vintage, London, 1996

♡ McHattie, Grace, *That's Cats*, David & Charles, Newton Abbot, 1991

♡ Morris, Desmond, *Catwatching*, Ebury Press, London, 1994

♡ Neville, Peter, *Cat Behaviour Explained*, Parragon Books, 1990

♡ Pitcairn, Richard & Pitcairn, Susan, *Dr Pitcairn's Complete Guide to Natural Health for Dogs & Cats*, Rodale Press, Philadelphia, 1982

♡ Tabor, Roger, *Understanding Cats*, David & Charles, Newton Abbot, 1995

♡ Taylor, David, *The Ultimate Cat Book*, Dorling Kindersley, London, 1989

Further study

In addition to the books listed above, you can now get videos, a cassette and CD-Rom to help you learn more about the remedies. All the following are available by mail order from the Bach Centre (see address on page 114).

♡ Cassette tape, *Getting to Know the Bach Flower Remedies* – side one gives you full descriptions of all 38 remedies, and side two gives you the chance to practise your knowledge in a series of exercises.

♡ Video, *The Light That Never Goes Out* – tells the story of Dr Bach's life and work.

♡ Video, *Bach Flower Remedies: A Further Understanding* – the trustees of the Bach Centre explain how to use the remedies.

♡ CD-Rom, *The Original Flower Remedies of Dr Bach* – a useful self-teach tool that presents the indications for the remedies and instructions for their use alongside excerpts from Dr Bach's own writings and video clips from the Bach Centre.

People all over the world run courses in using the remedies. Here is an overview of what is available:

♡ *Bach International Education Programme* courses are quality controlled by the Dr Edward Bach Foundation and run in many countries around the world. The Programme comprises three levels of training – level 1, level 2 and level 3 practitioner training. You can obtain more details from either the Bach Centre or Nelsons.

♡ *Correspondence courses* have a reputation for being over-priced and inaccurate, so be careful before parting with money. Any correspondence course that claims to equip you for professional practice should be treated with extreme caution. The Dr Edward Bach Foundation runs its own introductory correspondence course, recognised as equivalent to a Bach International Education Programme level 1 course. Contact the Bach Centre for details.

♡ *Approved courses* include approved introductory courses run by registered practitioners, plus special days on particular subjects. Every year there are courses run specifically for people who want to use the remedies to help animals. Places are limited, and applicants are expected to know all 38 remedies and to have attained a standard equivalent to having followed the official level 2 course. Contact the Bach Centre for more details.

♡ *Independent training* varies from short talks at local centres to full-scale courses costing hundreds of pounds. The quality and accuracy of teaching varies, so if possible look for a course run by a qualified registered practitioner. The Bach Centre may know of one near you.

Bach addresses

The Dr Edward Bach Centre

The Bach Centre is housed in Mount Vernon, the Victorian cottage that Dr Bach chose to be the centre of his work. The mother tinctures for the Bach Flower Remedies are still made there today using the same methods that Dr Bach used. You can visit the house and garden and there is a shop on site selling remedies and educational material. Callers can get free help and advice by letter, phone or email, or can be referred to trained practitioners who are registered with the Dr Edward Bach Foundation (see below).

Address: Mount Vernon, Bakers Lane, Sotwell, Wallingford, Oxon, OX10 0PZ, England
Tel: 00 44 (0) 1491 834678
Fax: 00 44 (0) 1491 825022
Email: bach@bachcentre.com
Website: http://www.bachcentre.com

The Dr Edward Bach Foundation

The Bach Centre set up the Dr Edward Bach Foundation in 1991 with the aim of training and registering practitioners. In partnership with the Education Department at A Nelson & Co (see below) the Foundation has helped set up a programme of training courses in many different parts of the world, including the USA, Canada, New Zealand, Spain, Brazil and Japan.

Address: Mount Vernon, Bakers Lane, Sotwell, Oxon, OX10 0PZ, England

Tel: 00 44 (0) 1491 834678

Fax: 00 44 (0) 1491 825022

Email: foundation@bachcentre.com

The Dr Edward Bach Healing Trust

The Trust, a registered charity, was originally set up in the 1950s to hold the house and garden at Mount Vernon in perpetuity. More recently it has taken on a more overtly charitable role, and helps to spread Dr Bach's system and message of self-help through donations of money and remedies.

Address: Mount Vernon, Bakers Lane, Sotwell, Oxon, OX10 0PZ, England

Tel: 00 44 (0) 1491 834678

Fax: 00 44 (0) 1491 825022

Email: trust@bachcentre.com

A Nelson & Co Ltd/Bach Flower Remedies Ltd

You can contact Nelsons for information on local availability of the remedies anywhere in the world. Through its Education Department, and in association with the Dr Edward Bach Foundation, Nelsons also runs the Bach International Education Programme.

Address: Broadheath House, 83 Parkside, London, SW19 5LP, England

Tel: 00 44 (0) 20 8780 4200
Fax: 00 44 (0) 20 8780 5871
Website: http://www.nelsons.co.uk

Other useful addresses

Australia

♡ Blue Cross Society Inc, Lot 9 Homestead Road,
Wonga Park, Victoria 3136. Tel: (03) 9722 1265.

♡ The Cat Protection Society of NSW, 103 Enmore Road,
Enmore, NSW 2042. Tel: (02) 9557 1011.

♡ Humane Society of Australia (NSW), 1/75 Pittwater Rd,
Manly, NSW 2095, Tel: (02) 9977 6303.

♡ Petcare Information and Advisory Service Australia Pty
Ltd, Level 13, Como, 644 Chapel Street, South Yarra,
Victoria 3141. Web site: www.petnet.com.au

♡ WSPA (World Society for the Protection of Animals)
Australia, 46 Nicholson Street, St Leonards, NSW 2065.
Tel: (2) 9901 5205. Email: kmjones@ozemail.com.au

Canada

♡ WSPA (World Society for the Protection of Animals)
Canada, 44 Victoria Street, Suite 1310, Toronto,
Ontario M5C 1Y2. Tel: +1 416 369 0044.
Email: wspacanada@compuserve.com

New Zealand

♡ Humane Society of NZ Inc, PO Box 29-060,
Greenswoods Corner, Auckland 1003.
Tel: (09) 630 0510.

♡ RNZSPCA (Inc), PO Box 15-349, New Lynn, Auckland.
Tel: (09) 827 6094.

UK

♡ APACHE (The Association for the Promotion of Animal Complementary Health Education), Archers Wood Farm, Coppingford Road, Sawtry, Huntingdon, Cambridgeshire, PE17 5XT. Tel: 07050 244196. E-mail: apache@avnet.co.uk Website: www.avnet.co.uk/~apache/

♡ British Homoeopathic Veterinary Association, Chinham House, Stanford-in-the-Vale, Faringdon, Oxfordshire, SN7 8NQ Tel: 01367 710324.

♡ Cats Protection, 17 Kings Road, Horsham, West Sussex, RH13 5PN. Tel: 01403 221900; helpline: 01403 221927.

♡ PDSA (People's Dispensary for Sick Animals), White Chapel, Priorslee, Telford, Shropshire, TF2 9PQ. Tel: 01952 290999.

♡ RSPCA (Royal Society for the Prevention of Cruelty to Animals), Causeway, Horsham, West Sussex, RH12 1HG. Tel: 01403 264181.

♡ WSPA (World Society for the Protection of Animals), 2 Langley Lane, London, SW8 1TJ. Tel: 020 7793 0540. Email: wspa@wspa.org.uk

USA

♡ American Pet Association, PO Box 7172, Boulder, CO 80306-7172. Tel: (888) 272 7387 or 800 APA PETS. Email: apa@apapets.com

♡ ASPCA (American Society for the Prevention of Cruelty to Animals), 424 East 92nd Street, New York, NY 10128-6804. Tel: (212) 876-7700. Website: www.aspca.org

♡ Humane Society of the United States, 2100 L St. NW, Washington, DC 20037. Website: www.hsus.org

♡ WSPA (World Society for the Protection of Animals) USA, 29 Perkins Street, PO Box 190, Boston, MA 02130. Tel: (617) 522 7000. Email: wspa@world.std.com

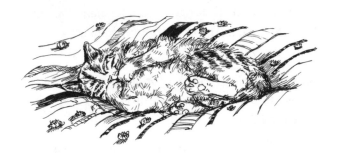

Index

ear problems 93–4
eating *see* food and feeding
eczema 89
Elm 11–12, 85
emotions ix, 3, 4, 52–68
encephalitis 56
encouragement 13, 58, 77, 95
energy 102, 105, 107, 108
    lack of 15, 30, 57, 75
enthusiasm 26, 40, 63, 75
    lack of 30, 40
environment 73–4
epiphora 91
evolution 3
exercise 65, 76, 97
Exotic Shorthairs 36
eye problems 91–2

faeces 66, 67, 84, 87
failure 2, 17
faintness 31
fasting 60, 98
fear ix, 5, 8, 14, 19, 34
    and aggression 52, 81
    and cat shows 84
    freezing reaction 21–2
    in humans 1, 74
    in kittens 70
    and separation 62, 80
    and specific causes 53, 55–6
feet 108
feline immunodeficiency virus 86
feline infectious anaemia 86
feline infectious enteritis 86
feline infectious peritonitis 86
feline leukaemia 86–7
feline upper respiratory tract
    disease 86, 92, 95
feline urological syndrome 66
fever 86
fighting 74, 78, 81
First Aid 47–52
fleas 90
'flu 86, 92, 95
fluid in abdomen 86
food and feeding 16, 57, 58–60,
    92, 95

and additives 62–3
after birth 77
and digestive problems 98–9
and newcomers to the house
    81
and obesity 96–7
see also appetite
food sources 72
frustration 26, 29, 44
fungal illness 94
fussiness 11, 41

genito-urinary problems 99–100
Gentian 2, 12, 44, 58, 95
    and despondency 80, 91
    and eating 92
    and eye problems 91
glaucoma 91
Gorse 13, 58, 80, 92, 95
grief 15, 24, 25, 44, 61–2
grooming 8, 82, 85, 99
    excessive 11, 63, 89, 90
guilt 20, 78
gums 95, 96

Hahnemann, Samuel 106
hair loss 84, 85, 89
hearing 93–4
Heather 13–14, 40, 41, 72, 95
    and attention-seeking 75, 82,
        87–8
    and self-pity 80, 82
heatstroke 51
herbal medicine 90, 105–6, 107
hesitation 17
Holly 14, 53, 73, 74, 82
homesickness 15
homoeopathy 1, 106–7
Honeysuckle 15, 45, 61, 83
    and adjustment 73, 80
hopelessness 13, 25, 58, 61
Hornbeam 15–16, 57, 69, 85
    and eating 92, 99
    and pregnancy and birth 76, 77
house move 79–80
hunters 34
hyperactivity 26, 62–3, 75, 84

panic 5, 8, 22, 31, 49, 77
parasites 90–1, 93, 94
patience 16
peace 105
pessimism 44, 58
Pine 20–1, 44, 78
Pitcairn, Richard (Dr) 24–5
plants 3–4, 103
play 5, 16, 62, 69–70, 87, 97
pneumonia 95
possessiveness 9–10, 46
pregnancy 60, 76
psychoneuroimmunology 4

Ragdoll cats 38
Red Chestnut 21, 44, 54, 60, 97
  and anxiety 56, 62, 70, 79
  and digestive problems 99
relaxation 103, 104, 105
reliability in cats 19, 41
repeat behaviour 9
rescue cats 82–3
Rescue Cream 33, 48, 50, 89, 92,
  95
rescue homes 24, 82–3
Rescue Remedy 31–3, 42, 48, 49,
  51, 77
  and burns 50
  calming effect 79, 84, 100
  and emergencies 88
  and eye problems 91
  and grief 61
  for kittens 70
  for rescue cats 82
  and respiratory problems 92,
    94, 95
  and stress 64, 68, 98
  and ticks 90
  and toothache 96
resentment 30–1
respiratory problems 86, 87, 92,
  94, 95
restlessness 17, 30, 61, 62, 88, 95
Rock Rose 14, 21–2, 31, 49, 56,
  77
  and fear 68, 74, 79, 83
Rock Water 22–3, 41

routine 19, 23
Russian Blue Cats 37

salivation 95
scent 65, 67, 78, 80–2, 91
Scleranthus 23–4, 40, 49, 57, 62,
  94
scratching 6, 9, 19, 58–9, 95
  uncontrolled 8, 94
scratching post 65
self-belief 7, 17
self-centredness 13–14, 40
self-confidence 2, 11, 12, 70, 75
  lack of 17, 73, 79
  and old age 85
  and rescue cats 83
  and spraying 64
self-control 31, 53, 77, 98
self-denial 2–23
self-injury 8, 94
self-pity 44, 80, 82, 88, 95
self-reliance 68
separation 61
seriousness 75
shame 11
shock 24–5, 31, 44, 70, 77
shorthaired cats 35–7
shyness 19, 39, 68, 70, 73
Siamese 26, 37
sickness 24, 49, 76, 86
skin problems 89
sleep 10, 40, 85, 95
  restless 4, 5, 29
sleeplessness 29, 62
smell 65, 67, 78, 80–2, 91
sneezing 86
solitude 73
Somali cats 38
spite 14, 73
spraying 5, 63–4, 78
Star of Bethlehem 24, 31, 44, 51,
  61
  and birth 69, 77
  and house move 79
  for kittens 70, 71
  for rescue cats 83
stings 47–8

123

strangers 10, 12, 72, 80–2
strays 79
street cats (Moggies) 36
stress 5, 45, 87, 95, 99
   and house move 79
   and hyperactivity 62, 63
   and toilet habits 64, 67
stropping 65–6
stud tail 89
submission 21, 28
sulking 30–1, 58
suspicion 74
Sweet Chestnut 25, 44, 58, 61

Tabby Longhairs 38
Tao philosophy 102
Taylor, Roger 52
teeth and teething 70, 84, 95
territory 52–3, 63–4, 67, 71, 79
   and stropping 65–6
terror 21–2, 31, 56, 74, 77
   and rescue cats 83
testicles 100
therapies, natural 101–9
thyroid problem 97
ticks 90
timidity 7, 19, 39, 70, 73
tiredness 15, 20, 85, 86
toilet habits 66–8, 84
tolerance 5–6, 41
Tortoiseshell Longhairs 38
toxoplasmosis 87
travel sickness 24, 49, 83
type remedies 39

urination 9, 63–4, 66–8, 78, 84,
   100
   and allergies 67

vaccines 1
vaginal discharge 99–100
Vervain 26, 40, 44, 54, 68
   and hyperactivity 63, 75, 84, 99
veterinary care 47, 48, 51, 58, 66,
   109

Vine 26–7, 39, 41, 53, 82
   and dominance 64, 72
viruses 86, 87, 92, 94
vomiting 24, 49, 76, 86, 98–9

Walnut 27–8, 44, 54, 62, 87
   and birth 78
   and change 49, 57, 61, 63, 64,
     68
     house move 79
     in relationships 30, 73, 81
     and rescue cats 83
     and stropping 66
   and kittens 69, 70, 71
   and obesity 97
   and old age 85
   and pregnancy 76
   and skin disorder 89
   and stress 49, 87
warts 89
water 42, 50–1, 98
Water Violet 28, 40, 54, 68, 71,
   98
   and loners 73, 82
weaning 70
weight loss 86, 87
White Chestnut 29, 44, 63
White Longhairs 38
Wild Oat 29
Wild Rose 30, 40, 57, 85, 95
   and birth 77
   and eating 92, 99
   and exercise 76
   and kittens 69
Willow 30, 44, 58, 91, 95
   and attention-seeking 82
   and discontent 75, 82
   and self-pity 80, 82, 88
Wilson, Edward O. 3
worms 90
worry 1, 25, 44, 79
   see also anxiety
wounds 48

yin and yang 102